MY MOTHER'S BREAST

MY MOTHER'S BREAST

Daughters Face Their Mothers' Cancer

LAURIE TARKAN

Taylor Publishing Company
Dallas, Texas

Published by Taylor Publishing Company
1550 West Mockingbird Lane
Dallas, Texas 75235
www.taylorpub.com

Library of Congress Cataloging-in-Publication Data

Tarkan, Laurie.
    My mother's breast : daughters face their mothers' cancer / Laurie
Tarkan.
        p.   cm.
    ISBN 0-87833-227-8
    1. Breast—Cancer—Psychological aspects. 2. Breast—Cancer—
Social aspects. 3. Mothers and daughters. I. Title.
RC280.B8T36   1998
362.1'9699449—dc21   99-12047
                                                    CIP

Printed in the United States of America
10 9 8 7 6 5 4 3 2 1

In memory of
Myrna Lindenberg Tarkan
(1936–1974)

For
Stuart Earl Tarkan

CONTENTS

FOREWORD

Kathryn M. Kash, PhD

*F*or the past ten years I have provided psychological counseling for women whose mothers, grandmothers, sisters, and even daughters have had breast cancer. More than three-fourths of these women had mothers with breast cancer, and many of their mothers succumbed to the disease. Women at increased risk for breast cancer, because of their family histories, are often emotionally distressed and unable to express the wide range of emotions they feel about their relative's cancer. These women frequently remain silent because they feel they cannot talk to anyone, and more important, they think their feelings are not normal. Women whose mothers developed breast cancer often suffer the greatest.

Over the course of this past decade I have found it both personally and professionally rewarding to help women become proactive in their health behaviors, particularly as they relate to breast cancer. In 1988 I began to explore the distress issues of women with family histories of breast cancer and found that 27 percent had levels of anxiety and depression consistent with a need for psychological counseling. Some women's levels of distress were as high as women who had endured and survived Leukemia and Hodgkin's disease. Through the initial research I did on the psychological issues for these women, counseling strategies emerged that women thought would be most useful for them. The popular request was a group intervention, a forum to openly express feelings of anxiety, fear of disease, vulnerability, anger, powerlessness over breast cancer development, guilt, and isolation and loneliness. In these groups of eight to ten women, handing out written material is extremely important, as it provides concrete information in a clear, concise, and articulate manner about the most salient aspects of breast cancer prevention and treatment, genetic issues, lifestyle behaviors, and stress management. One of the articles that has been given out for the past four years is Laurie Tarkan's "How Daughters Face Their Mothers' Breast Cancer," which was published in the October 1994 issue of *McCall's* magazine. Since then, women have been reading it as part of the material for the group session on stress management and coping with being at increased risk for breast cancer. This article has indeed proved invaluable for the daughters of women with breast cancer. For them, it confirms many of the feelings that have been buried inside them for a long time, sometimes as long as twenty years.

All the above exemplifies the need for the chapters in this book. To date, this is the only book that explores the multitude of psychological issues mentioned above that women with mothers with breast cancer think about and cope with almost daily. Reading this book, women will find at least one, and perhaps more than one, woman they can identify with, and thus have the needed validation for their range of feelings about breast cancer. The content of each chapter is quite rich and will provide women with insight into themselves and their mothers. The chapter on a mom who survived breast cancer is essential reading, as it allows daughters to realize that women do survive breast cancer and go on to lead full and meaningful lives as survivors. This chapter also describes a mother's concern about passing on the legacy of breast cancer. All the emotional issues that women have faced are covered in this book, from personal stories to the section on getting help, and more specifically, how to live without fear.

Laurie Tarkan has provided in-depth coverage of the struggles, the fears, the sadness, and the hopes of women facing the threat of breast cancer. It will be welcomed by daughters of women with breast cancer and by women who have family histories of breast cancer, as well as by women who are breast cancer survivors. The emotional issues, which are often gut-wrenching, are the main purpose of this book and are explored in a most sensitive manner. I would highly recommend *My Mother's Breast* to all women who want to cope with their worries about breast cancer and move forward with their lives.

Kathryn M. Kash, PhD
Director, Psychological Services
Strang Cancer Prevention Center
Assistant Professor of Psychology in Psychiatry
The New York Hospital–Cornell Medical Center

PREFACE

*W*hen I was an editorial assistant at *Self* magazine ten years ago, my company held a blood drive, so like most conscientious employees, I went down to the conference room, lay down on a portable bed, and offered up my arm. The nurse cleansed my forearm, jabbed it, adjusted the sac, and let me be. But a sac of blood takes a few minutes to fill. As I waited, tears started rolling down my cheeks. The nurse, noticing my situation, came over and asked what hurt. "It doesn't hurt," I said. "It's just something sad I thought of." As I lay there with my arm out and a tube stuck in it, I thought of my mother as she was when I went to the hospital to visit her when I was ten years old. I remember her lying in the hospital bed with her arm by her side and IV tubes snaking out of her wrist, rising up to a couple of limpid pouches hanging on a tall metal stand. I was frightened by those tubes, invading her body like the disease itself. I was devastated to see my precious mom so weak and sick, and at the mercy of those tubes.

I remember very little of the time before February 26, 1974, the day my mother, Myrna Tarkan, died. I was only eleven years old. Most of these memories, like the hospital scene, are sad or frightening. I have memories of her being too weak to get out of bed or contending with one annoying symptom or another. That could be the result of a morbid selective memory on my part, but it could be the result of the way my mother's illness was handled in my family. My mother and father went to great lengths to protect me and my older sister, Gail, from knowing the extent of her illness. My father believed that the trauma of knowing that our mother was dying would be worse for us than the consequences of not knowing. But my mother kept the truth from us for another reason. She thought that she would live. She had been diagnosed with a rare liver disorder ten years before she died. One internist told her she could live a relatively long life with the help of drugs to moderate her symptoms. Another internist, fresh out of medical school, said to my twenty-seven-year-old mother, "What are you worried about? You have another ten good years ahead of you." That made my mother cry.

The young internist was callous but prophetic, though my mother chose to align herself with the older physician's prognosis. She was optimistic about her life. Like many patients with life-threatening diseases, she did not see herself as a dying person; she saw herself fighting the disease with whatever medicine had to offer, ever hopeful that the next treatment would cure her. She always pushed forward, despite pain, fatigue, fever, and other symptoms. She continued teaching at the local high school, pursuing her doctorate in education, keeping up an active social life, and raising Gail and me. She didn't think she was dying so she didn't think she needed to burden us with the scary details of her illness. Though my mother was sick on and off for many years, and very sick the last two years of her life, her death came as a shock to me and my older sister. We were not prepared.

Sometimes I feel that it was not my mother's illness and death that had the greatest impact on my life, affecting my relationships with people and my sense of security in the world, but rather the silence around that illness. That silence left me with more than the loss of my mother. I lost her without ever being able to say goodbye, or being able to say anything meaningful. We never had that conversation in which my mother would tell me how much she loved me or what a wonderful little girl I was, or how I would succeed in life, or simply that she did not want to leave me. A child does not assume these things; a child does not infer; a child needs to hear the words to know that they are true. So I was left to wonder about these things all my life.

As much as I wonder about her feelings toward me, I wonder about who she was. I was too young to experience her as a person, with all her quirks and vulnerabilities and lovable and not so lovable traits. The knowledge I have about my mother, the woman I envision as Mom, has been cobbled together from the stories I've heard, photographs I've seen, and my own small bank of memories. The image is minimal at best, a few poignant stories and a list of traits—funny, vivacious, warm, athletic, intelligent, beautiful. She was a feminist who loved the theater, the ballet, antiques, and clothes. It all fills me with great pride, and a great sadness, selfishly for what I missed.

My regret of not knowing my mother has become more cogent since I embarked on this book. During my interviews with daughters, I was struck by a feeling I wasn't expecting. I envied the time those daughters who had their mothers in their teenage years and in their twenties and thirties and the intimate mother-daughter bond many had described, a bond unlike all others in life. But in writing this book, I have learned more about my mother. I learned because I was compelled for the sake of the book to seek out more information about her life, her sickness, and her death. It forced me to broach the subject of my mother's illness to my father and for us to speak at length about it for the first time. Those conversations have brought us even closer. I also learned about my mother through the stories I heard from mothers and daughters. These stories have given me insight into what my own mother must have experienced during her illness and what I, as a young child, went through.

My mother died of a rare liver disorder. In interviewing the women for this book, I felt I should apologize because she didn't have breast cancer. It would have made more sense for me to write this book if she had. As a health writer, I have written on different medical and psychology topics, many of which do not resonate with me personally. But one day I was speaking with a social worker at Cancer Care, Inc., an organization that offers social services and support for women with cancer, and she mentioned that she occasionally counsels daughters of breast cancer patients. Given my own personal background, I immediately took interest in the topic and wrote an article about these daughters for *McCall's* magazine, which did touch me deeply. The stories I heard from the daughters I interviewed seemed to reflect my own experiences. The daughters made me cry for them and for myself. They also made me laugh and left me feeling stronger and more hopeful. The article won an award, the Rose Kushner Award for Writing Achievement in the Field of Breast Cancer. Rose Kushner was a journalist who, back in the 1970s, was one of the first breast cancer patients to speak out about the disease and the need for better early detection and better treatments. The award made me realize that this is a topic that needs more attention, so I began to think about writing a book.

I embarked on this book as I approached the age of thirty-seven, my mother's age when she died. I was afraid that this endeavor would dig up some deep feelings of fear and grief that were buried in my unconscious a long time ago. I was afraid that every story I heard would bring me to tears. To some degree, I haven't been my lighthearted self during this enterprise. But I haven't been a wreck either. The reason I could hold it together was that these stories of daughters aren't all doom and gloom. Many are warm and inspiring, and sometimes humorous; they are about loss and fear but also about courage and love, mother love and the importance of mother-daughter relationships. Many of the daughters have learned from the cancer experience, becoming better people and living richer lives because of it.

For me, my mother's sickness and her death have both given and taken. They have given me access to the extremes of the emotional world—profound sadness and an exhilarating joy. They have acquainted me with grief at a young age, but have given me a deep sense of compassion for others. They have made me feel alone, but have enabled me to move through my life independently. They have made me feel like an outsider, left out of the normal currents of life (an eleven-year-old dressing up to go to her mother's funeral is no longer like the other kids who are dressing down for a game of kickball). But being outside has forced me to take unconventional and ultimately rewarding courses in life. My mother's sickness and death have introduced me to my own mortality at a pre-adolescent age, yet I've responded by developing an adventurous, risk-taking spirit and a giddy gusto for life as well as the determination to live the rest of my life happily. Mostly, I've pushed myself to go beyond what feels comfortable, motivated perhaps by the need for approval from the one woman who is no longer here to dispense it. In pushing myself, I have achieved more than I thought I could, more than I would have had I not seen those tubes coming out of my mother's wrist when I was a little girl.

ACKNOWLEDGMENTS

I am deeply grateful to the daughters and mothers who showed great courage in sharing their stories for this book. They spoke with honesty and candor and with the sole purpose and hope of helping other women who may find themselves venturing up this difficult trail after them. They are Caleen, Cynthia, Felicia, Jennifer, Jill, Judy, Julie, Karen, Kathie, Lauren, Lisa, Marcia, Mickey, Sandy, Stephanie, Sunshine, and Suzanne and others who chose to remain anonymous. I am also grateful to the many other daughters, sisters, and mothers who talked to me, whose stories I could not include, but whose thoughts and experiences are intricately woven into the fabric of the book.

My deepest thanks belong to my father, Stuart Tarkan, who, after the death of my mother, filled the roles of both mother and father for my sister and me. He is a generous and caring man, my oldest and best friend, who has encouraged me, consoled me, guided me, taught me, and most recently has endured my difficult questions about my mother's illness for this book. I also owe thanks to my husband, Andrew, whose love and support kept me going through this emotionally difficult endeavor.

This book would not exist without my agents: Connie Clausen was the first to understand my vision for the book, a vision that she sharpened with her insight and nourished with her encouragement. I was fortunate to have worked with her and known her before her sudden death in September 1997. I continued the project with her associate, Stedman Mays, whose warmth, enthusiasm, and humor have kept me inspired and confident through the writing process. From the beginning, my editor, Camille Cline, believed in the importance of this book and its contribution to filling the void for daughters. I am deeply grateful to her for helping me to achieve my vision.

Christine Many, my research assistant, worked after hours to help with the medical research. Lynn Ermann and Hilary Macht took time out of their own journalism schedule to read my early drafts, and offered insightful and creative feedback. My mentors, Lynne Cusack and Lorraine Daigneault, two brilliant and generous women, have guided me at different stages of my journalism career and have given me valuable advice on this book.

I'm grateful to the following people who provided their expertise and knowledge on the subjects of mother-daughter relationships, living with sickness, death and dying, and breast cancer. They are Evelyn Bassoff, Barbara Bernhardt, Margaret Burke, Bruce Compas, Robert T. Croyle, Marguerite Eng, Sydney Ey, Sandra Haber, Hester Hill, Roberta Hufnagel, Christina Pozo Kaderman, Kathryn Kash, Caryn Lerman, Frances Marcus Lewis, Sue Miesfeldt, Julianne Oktay, June Peters, Adrienne Ressler, Gladys Rosenthal, Allison Ross, Pat Spicer, Jill Stopfer, David Wellisch, and the women at the Susan G. Komen Foundation, Cancer Care, Inc., and SHARE.

INTRODUCTION

$\int$ ix days after her mother died of breast cancer, Lauren Piskin, thirty-three years old at the time and the mother of two young girls, found a lump the size of a marble in her own breast and was certain that it was malignant. Lauren had watched her mother suffer a long illness and watched her mother die, and she was sure that she would follow in her footsteps. She staggered through the next few days of doctors' visits and diagnostic tests, already grieving her own life. When the results of the biopsy came back, her own dire predictions proved false. The lump was benign. Lauren would live. The biopsy, however, left a small scar on Lauren's right breast, an indelible reminder of the disease, a mark of the macabre legacy her mother left her.

If you have been handed down this legacy, if your mother has been diagnosed with cancer, this book is for you. You are not the patient yourself, and you cannot presume to be going through what your mother is, but you struggle with it in your own way. It is a harrowing experience for a young woman to watch a mother threatened by any serious illness, and it is especially distressing when the illness is breast cancer. Although tens of thousands of women survive breast cancer every year, and strides have been made toward its diagnosis and treatment, the word *cancer* still evokes fears of disfigurement, pain, and death. Maybe in five years, or ten, it won't. For now, the diagnosis still comes with the prospect and the fear of losing mother, which is, for most of us, one of the greatest losses we will face in life. A mother's diagnosis of cancer, however, comes with another burden. It plucks you out of the general population and places you in a group of high-risk women. Because of the widely publicized genetic link of breast cancer, you face the inescapable question,

"Will I be next?" I interviewed more than seventy women for this book, women of all ages and from across the country, and most of the daughters felt certain that they knew the answer.

"The impact of breast cancer comes from two directions," explains Roberta Hufnagel, PhD, a New York City psychotherapist who counsels breast cancer patients and their daughters, and who is a breast cancer survivor herself. "First, you have the threat of losing this unbelievably important person who is almost a lifeline to you. Second, because you are so identified with your mother, it's almost as if you're losing yourself, too. It feels as though what is happening to mother is happening to you," says Hufnagel.

Daughters try to cope with the crisis of their mothers' illness, they try not to focus on their fears, they try to take care of their mother, to be strong for her and to hold out hope. They try to put their differences behind them and push their concerns for their own body and their own life to the back of their mind. But it's difficult, not only because they're filled with worry and stress, feeling as though a tornado has spun through their life, tossing everything into disarray, but because this crisis is staged within the context of an already complex mother-daughter relationship and because they have lost more than they may realize.

Breast cancer disrupts the natural order of life. We all know, in the deep recesses of our minds, that one day we will care for our ailing mother and one day we will mourn our mother's death. But we banish the thought. Healthy denial preserves our sanity by keeping us from acknowledging this frightening prospect until we're older, more established with our own families and perhaps beginning to feel the tug of aging ourselves. Breast cancer, however, often makes daughters face this inevitability early in life, much too early. "You lose your innocence as a result of being dealt this blow. You lose that normal expectation that your mother will live to a reasonably ripe old age and that you will live to a ripe old age," says Hufnagel. We all go through life with a basic assumption that our parents are going to protect us and be strong for us and be there as a safe haven if we get sick or end a relationship or get fired from a job. We can always run home. "When you don't have healthy parents, it changes your own sense of power and invulnerability and confidence in the world," adds Allison Ross, PhD, a psychologist who is in private practice in New York City.

This is something many will have to face one day, but it is more difficult if it happens when a woman is young, in her teens, twenties, or thirties, when she still has the important rites of passage ahead of her, those big moments in life when mother is expected to be there, looking on proudly and guiding her through. Among the daughters I interviewed for this book—sixteen whose stories I tell in full—many were approaching milestones when their mothers were diagnosed. "It came at a real critical time when I was in the midst of planning a wedding," says Caleen, a thirty-four-year-old public relations manager from Houston, who was twenty-nine when her mother was diagnosed (see *Making a Difference*). "I was seven months pregnant with my first child," says Lauren, who was twenty-seven when her mother got cancer. "I was scheduled to fly to San Francisco to give my first major presentation at a big national conference," says Jennifer, twenty-nine, a political scientist living in Baltimore (see *Depression and Fear*). "I found out the cancer had spread to her lungs a few days before my college graduation," says Sunshine, a twenty-two-year-old blond from Las Vegas (see *Mothering Mom*). Cancer transforms every one of these experiences.

Likewise, among the women I interviewed, many daughters were at an emotional crossroad with their mother: a daughter who was rebelling against her mother in an effort to become her own person, one who was struggling to free herself from a mother's dominant grip, and one who was just beginning to know her mother as an adult and to relate to her as a friend. Your mother may be your best friend, she may be your biggest critic, she may fill you with admiration or make you cringe in embarrassment, she may encourage you to do great things and frustrate you to no end, but a mother, even one who is flawed, is tantamount to your being.

Each year about 181,000 women in the United States are diagnosed with breast cancer and about 43,800 women die of the disease. All told, over a ten-year period, almost two million women are diagnosed, and for each woman diagnosed, her daughters, sisters, aunts, nieces, and mothers are directly and indirectly affected by her disease.

Much is known of the ordeal a woman with cancer goes through, and many books have been written about what she, as a patient, can expect physically and emotionally. But little is known about what a daughter goes through emotionally, and little has been written. "There is a huge population of daughters, millions and millions, and it is the most ignored population in terms of the impact that cancer has on the family," says David Wellisch, PhD, professor of medical psychology at the University of California at Los Angeles, who stumbled onto the plight of daughters when he realized how anxious his breast cancer patients became when they spoke about their daughters. Things are just beginning to change for daughters. Researchers who are interested in what keeps high-risk women from seeking appropriate preventive care, and mammography, have been delving into their emotional lives. Likewise, with the advent of genetic testing, researchers have begun to look at what motivates some women to get tested to see if they have inherited one of the gene mutations that have been linked with an increased risk of breast cancer. Moreover, they are studying what happens to women emotionally when they get their results.

The preliminary research, a dozen or so studies on the psychological effects of having a mother with breast cancer, have shown encouraging results. Most daughters are not necessarily more depressed than the average woman. This is especially true for women whose mothers have survived cancer. However, daughters do tend to have more intrusive thoughts about breast cancer during their day-to-day lives; they are more anxious and worried and have more sleep problems than the average person. If the daughters are adolescents or young adults still living at home, they have above average levels of depression and anxiety, according to Bruce Compas, PhD, psychologist at the University of Vermont, who has focused his research on the effect of a parent's cancer on her adolescent children. The main reason for their distress, Compas's studies conclude, is not so much the fear of losing mom, but the burden of taking on many more responsibilities than they should have at that age, which changes their day to day life drastically.

Although every daughter's experience with her mother's cancer is unique and every girl and woman emerges from it differently, I did hear several common themes repeated by the daughters I interviewed. Thirty-seven-year-old Karen, from Illinois, expresses what many daughters agree was the most difficult aspect of this. "The worst part was when she was in pain. To see her hurt like that was ripping me apart inside. There was nothing I could do to stop the hurt." Watching helplessly as a loved one suffers from a pain that you cannot control is one of the most devastating things to bear. Universally, daughters also expressed a fear of their mothers dying, even those daughters who intellectually knew their mother had an excellent chance of survival because the cancer was detected early. Furthermore, daughters, true to their female role as nurturers, were often called upon to provide emotional support for their mothers, their siblings, and even for their fathers. Although many fathers were supportive, just as many, according to their daughters, "couldn't handle it" or "were a wreck." Lastly, many daughters, even women in their teenage years, expressed sadness that they had to reverse roles with their mother and physically and emotionally become their mother's mother.

From here, the stories veer off in many directions. Some daughters deal with their mothers' cancer with optimism and hope; some fall into a deep depression; some drop everything in their lives, including their own husbands, to take care of their mothers; some avoid their mother while she's ill; some turn a bad relationship with mother into a wonderful one; some make life-transforming decisions for themselves, like getting a divorce or deciding to have a baby; some become exceedingly anxious about their own risk of breast cancer; and some, in honor of their mother, have become hard-working volunteers for the breast cancer cause.

The ways a daughter handles her mother's cancer are as varied as the girls and women themselves and the families in which they were raised. It depends largely on the person, whether she is optimistic or pessimistic, carefree or worried, emotional or even-keeled. It depends on many variables—how advanced the cancer is, how well her mother responds to treatment, her mother's coping skills, how good or poor the mother-daughter relationship is, how openly the family communicates, whether there is any dysfunction in the home like alcoholism, how supportive her father and other siblings are, and how involved the daughter becomes in the care of her mother.

Perhaps most significant, though, a daughter's reaction depends on whether the cancer metastasized and her mother has died. The experience of a daughter whose mother dies is vastly different from one whose mother survives. David Wellisch found that when a mother dies, daughters are more likely to have reversed the mother-daughter roles and cared for their mothers in the final stages of their illness; they are more likely to have altered their long-range plans in life because of the cancer; they believe their mothers were more distraught about breast cancer than other daughters whose mothers survived; and they are left with higher levels of anxiety for their own risk of cancer.

Indeed, many daughters of women who had advanced breast cancer are so fearful of getting cancer themselves that they say things like, "I feel like a walking time bomb," or they'll start a sentence with, "When I get breast cancer . . . " as if it were *fait accompli*. Witnessing their mothers endure the symptoms of advanced cancer has scared them to death. If they are mourning their mother's death, their grief serves to heighten the fear. "When you ask daughters what their risk is, many overestimate it," says Kathryn Kash, PhD, chief psychologist at the Strang Cancer Prevention Center at the New York Hospital–Cornell Medical Center, one of the original researchers of daughters of breast cancer patients. "Some say 80 percent, some say 150 percent, which is mathematically impossible. They are so convinced it's their destiny." Many daughters have no doubt that their family has a mutation in one of two genes, BRCA1 or BRCA2, that have been linked to a greatly increased risk of breast cancer. The reality is that only about 5 percent of women with breast cancer have these mutations and only 15 to 25 percent have a family history of breast cancer. In fact, to dispel another misconception, for many women with a family history of cancer, their actual lifetime risk rises very little over the average woman's risk, a couple of percentage points, and some even maintain the same risk as those in the general population, one in nine at age eighty-five. But try telling that to a daughter whose mother died of breast cancer; she'll laugh in your face and accuse you of trying to put one over on her.

Daughters feel so certain of their fate, however wrong it may be, because it's natural to believe that whatever happens to your mother's body is going to happen to yours. "Every daughter—of healthy and sick women alike—feels a strong identification with her mother's body and a sense of continuity between her and her mother. She knows she's made out of the same cloth," says Evelyn Bassoff, PhD, a mother and a psychologist from Boulder, Colorado, who has written extensively on mother-daughter relationships. With breast cancer, these irrational feelings are affirmed and heightened because of the genetic link. Many women spend their entire life worrying about reaching the age that their mothers were diagnosed, fearing that this is precisely the age when they'll get cancer, too. This feeling that what happens to mother will happen to me works to the advantage of daughters whose mothers are survivors. They too believe they will get breast cancer, but they are often less grim about their own future, "knowing" that they will survive as their mothers did. As Andrea, a thirty-one-year-old graduate student from St. Paul, Minnesota, whose mother is a survivor, puts it, "In some ways, I dread it more now because I know statistically I'm more likely to get it, but in some ways, I dread it less, because I saw my mom go through it and survive it fine."

At Risk and Alone

When David Wellisch began his research on daughters, it was the easiest population he's ever recruited. Within three days of placing an advertisement in a local suburban newspaper, he had almost 400 women willing to participate—more than enough for his research. They responded because they had nowhere else to turn. "I felt like nobody else really understood, not my friends or my boyfriend," says Laura, a twenty-nine-year-old psychologist, echoing the sentiments of other daughters. "Nobody understood the kind of blow this was." When Sue, thirty-six years old, a book editor in New York City whose mother was two months away from dying of breast cancer, told her boss that she was going through a hard time, her boss, a woman, said, "Sue, we all have problems." Daughters shoulder a great emotional and often physical burden, and they usually carry it silently and alone, without advice, without comfort, and without support.

"When I started doing research with daughters, I found women who were exceedingly distressed about their situations and who had been prevailed upon to provide a lot of support and attention and had gotten very little of their own," says Wellisch. The mother has resources, like support groups—both live or on the Internet—as well as the team of health care professionals that is treating her, and there are even support groups for spouses of women with cancer. But there is virtually nothing for daughters.

The group has been overlooked because they are not quite patients themselves. "We have ignored this population, in part because the breast cancer movement is made up of survivors and this is an issue that may be hard for that group to look at," says Julianne Oktay, MS, professor of social work at the University of Maryland and co-author of *Breast Cancer in the Life Course.* "It's hard because the stories of the suffering of their daughters are extremely difficult for mothers to hear and may make them feel additionally guilty that they've done something terrible to their child," adds Oktay, who is now focusing her research on daughters. The stories in this book may be hard for mothers to read.

By the same token, many daughters feel they have to stifle their concerns and fears about themselves because they believe that people would consider such feelings self-centered in the face of their mothers' plights. After all, their mothers are the patients, not them. Some women also feel they have to be strong, upbeat, and optimistic for their mothers and their family, so they don't allow themselves to cry or to feel sad. Even many of the most educated daughters and those with good support systems simply do not know how to deal with the fear, the stress, the grief, the sadness, the guilt, and all the rest of the feelings they have toward their mothers' illnesses and their own risk. "Daughters are usually amazed at what feelings are buried that come out," says June Peters, MS, a senior genetic counselor at the University of Pittsburgh, who counsels high-risk women seeking risk assessment or genetic testing. A daughter simply may not feel comfortable sharing these complex emotions with her usual confidantes—particularly if her confidante is her mother.

When daughters don't talk about their feelings, they can get overwhelmed by them. Keeping in their emotions can lead to anxiety, depression, and anger, which can cause a daughter to make negative choices in her life and in her role in her mother's illness and recovery. It can hamper her ability to enjoy her own relationships and her own life. Jennifer, of Baltimore, became depressed after her mother's cancer metastasized, spread to other organs in her body. "I'm of the opinion that any activity that's not going to extend my mother's life isn't worth doing," she states. Karen, who has kept her feelings to herself, says, "I walk around angry. I take it out on people I shouldn't. I'm mad my mom's not here and that nobody could do anything to keep her here." Perhaps most worrisome, if daughters don't seek out someone to talk to, their fear may intensify to the point that they are afraid to seek the appropriate preventive medical care, such as regular breast exams and mammography. As Karen admits, "I hardly ever do breast self-exams. I don't want to feel my breasts because I'm scared of what I might find." They may also miss the opportunity to make lifestyle changes that may reduce their risk of breast cancer, such as exercising more, eating healthier foods, and avoiding alcohol.

Many of the daughters I interviewed for this book seemed surprised and relieved that I was asking how they fared during their mothers' cancer. For some, our conversations alone helped them work through some of their unresolved feelings about their mothers' illness. Being asked to delve deeper into their feelings was revealing to them, and voicing them was therapeutic. Some women realized they had feelings they had never known, and some went back to talk to their mothers about things they hadn't discussed. After speaking with many women, I selected sixteen whose stories seem to capture the different feelings and themes that arise for daughters.

Lauren, the mother of two, who had her own cancer scare, so identified with her mother that when her mother got cancer, she felt as if she were going through cancer herself (see *Friends and Foes*). Felicia, on the other hand, a forty-three-year-old poet and professor of English, had a troubled relationship with her mother and felt a sudden urgency to make things right after her mother was diagnosed. Sunshine, the post-grad from Las Vegas, and twenty-year-old Jill from Long Island, New York, both became their mothers' caretakers and dealt with the stress of a role reversal at a young age (see *Mothering Mom*). Suzanne and Lisa, two close sisters living in Boston, were glued to their mother's side from the moment of diagnosis through her last chemotherapy treatment (see *Sisters Sticking Together*). Kathie, forty-six, a costume designer from San Francisco, was diagnosed with breast cancer, as her mother was, but Kathie handled her own cancer much better than she handled her mother's (see *My Mother, My Self*). Nineteen-year-old Stacey (name has been changed) was a troubled teenager whose rebelliousness intensified when her mother was diagnosed (see *Adolescent Angst*). Kelly (name has been changed), from Canada, who was only eleven years old when her mother was diagnosed, and Julie, thirty-five, a therapist living in Southern California, both developed body image problems because of their fear of breast cancer (see *Adolescent Angst*). Stephanie, a thirty-five-year-old hair colorist from New York City, was estranged from her mother but finally came home when her mother's cancer metastasized (see *Anger and Love*). Jennifer, the political scientist from Baltimore, fell into a depression and has put her life on hold as she awaits the outcome of her mother's treatment (see *Depression and Fear*). Judy, forty-one, a marriage, family, and child counselor from Northern California, became so fearful of cancer that she decided to have a prophylactic mastectomy, the controversial procedure in which a high-risk woman's healthy breasts are removed preventively (see *Depression and Fear*). Caleen, the public relations pro, and Marcia, a forty-three-year-old New Yorker who works in international development, both became activists for the breast cancer cause. Cynthia, thirty-one, a commodities broker on Wall Street, tells a story about the personal growth that occurred as she was dealing with her mother's illness.

The stories of these women of all ages and from all parts of the country, presented with complete honesty and candor, will provide insight into your own experience. You may, as you read, feel some relief from the anxieties and feelings that have weighed you down. Maybe this book will motivate you to reach out to other daughters or to seek appropriate medical care and counseling if it's something you need. As Julianne Oktay puts it, "We need to pay more attention to how to make this experience less painful and more meaningful for daughters." I hope this book will do that for you.

Part One

DAUGHTERS' STORIES

1

FRIENDS AND FOES

"It's not good to be so attached—because when illness comes, it is devastating. It is like losing a limb."

Lauren Piskin, 38

LAUREN PISKIN
SYOSSET, NEW YORK

*B*efore breast cancer, Lauren Piskin never questioned the attachment that she felt toward her mother, and indeed, she felt lucky to consider her mother, Joan, her best friend. Lauren and Joan, though separated by a generation, were two of a kind, possessing the type of mystical connection that twins often report. They talked alike, they could finish each other's sentences, they had the same mannerisms, the same high-pitched laugh, the same lithe bodies, and they were both warm and open, the kind of people you'd feel comfortable confiding in. Even Lauren's passion for figure skating was an echo of her mother's schooling in ballet. As Lauren passed through her twenties, her feelings, her thoughts, her psyche and identity were still entwined with her mother's.

As a young girl, Lauren believed that she was one of the lucky ones. She grew up happy, in a quiet suburban neighborhood in Jericho, Long Island, with a mother who doted on her family. "My mother spent her whole life involved with me and

my brother, but she was almost obsessed with me," recalls
Lauren, now thirty-eight years old. She traces their bond back to
the days when she began figure skating. Her mother would shut-
tle Lauren back and forth from early-morning skating lessons,
school, after-school lessons, and competitions. The demanding
schedule forced them together for a large part of each day, but
Joan's support went beyond playing chauffeur. She anticipated—
and took care of—all her daughter's needs.

While the mother-daughter bond is naturally strong, most
girls and their mothers eventually jiggle it loose. Mothers try to
encourage independence, and girls rebel in various ways when
they struggle to achieve their individuality. Lauren never did.
When she got married, she moved twenty minutes away from
home and called her mother four or five times a day. Her mother
was always there to help. "If I had a problem, I'd tell her and
she'd give me the answer and I would accept it. My mother
always coped for me. She was my strength," says Lauren. But
with hindsight, Lauren admits, "It's not good to be so attached—
because when illness comes, it is devastating. It is like losing
a limb."

Lauren remembers in vivid detail the day her parents rushed
home, cutting short their vacation, because her mother felt two
lumps in her breast. Lauren was twenty-seven years old at the
time and seven months pregnant with her first child. She and her
husband had been living with her parents because their own
home was being renovated. "I remember their faces. They were
panic-stricken." They were worried because less than a year
before, Joan had found a lump and had a mammogram, an X ray
of the breast, but the test didn't detect anything suspicious. Now
the family was afraid the mammogram missed something. "We
didn't question the mammogram or tell her to get a second opinion because we were all so relieved," Lauren recalls. But the new
mammogram confirmed their worst fear: Joan, at the age of fifty,
had breast cancer which seemed to be advanced. Cancer was also
detected in eight lymph nodes, a sign that cancerous cells had
probably migrated to other parts of the body. Everything was a
crisis from that moment on.

"After they got the news, I remember my father pacing in

the garage crying. My mother was in the bathroom crying hysterically, saying she wanted to see her children grow old, to see her son get gray on his temples, her grandchildren get married," says Lauren.

Joan had both breasts removed in a procedure called a bilateral modified mastectomy, and then she underwent chemotherapy, in which potent cancer-killing drugs are given in a pill or intravenously once every two or three weeks for about six months. Because of the potency of these drugs, after each treatment, women typically suffer from fatigue, nausea, and vomiting; over the course of the treatment, many lose their hair. The family embraced Joan during this difficult time, and closed themselves off from the rest of the world. Lauren never left her mother's side. She didn't talk to her friends, didn't answer the phone, and even shut out her husband. "It was my mother, me, my father and brother, and that was it," recalls Lauren. "At first I couldn't get hold of myself. I could barely find my way through each day. You are almost your mother living through the pain. You cannot even make the separation. I identified so much with my mother."

Lauren's reaction is not unusual. There is such a strong identification physically between mother and daughter that many daughters believe whatever happens to their mothers is going to happen to them, says psychologist Evelyn Bassoff. When there is still that childlike identification with mother, as Lauren had, a daughter can feel as if there is no way of separating herself from what her mother is experiencing.

While the family was still in crisis mode, Lauren gave birth to her first child, Rachel. "I don't know if the elation of having a baby could be any greater than what we all felt," says Lauren. For her mother, though, it was bittersweet. "My mom spent most of my labor in the hospital bathroom throwing up and running a temperature from the chemotherapy. When they wheeled Rachel out to her, she was lying on the floor with my brother, praying she would be strong enough to stand up to see her granddaughter," recalls Lauren. Soon after the birth, the family got more good news: Joan's cancer was eradicated. So the family returned to a relatively normal life, with Lauren once again turning to her mother for advice and support in raising her child.

But two and a half years later, during a routine X ray of Joan's lungs, a shadow was detected. Further tests confirmed that her cancer had metastasized to her lungs and liver. When cancer spreads to other organs, chances of survival drop dramatically—the five-year survival rate, the standard measure of the effectiveness of treatment, is about 22 percent. For Lauren's family, the whole cycle of panic, fear, treatments, and pain started again, and that's when Lauren realized that she hadn't done a very good job at emotionally separating from her mother. Joan began taking the chemotherapy drug Taxol, which doctors say helped keep her alive for six years, far longer than they had predicted. But they were years of turmoil for Lauren and her family.

> *It's almost like my life for six years had been stop and hold, stop and hold. I pushed my husband away from the beginning. The relationship with him came second, or third, since I had two daughters by then. I was angry at my husband a lot because I didn't think he understood since his parents are healthy. Luckily, he was very close to my mother, which I think saved our marriage. When I look back, I realize how extremely supportive he was through all those years. But I couldn't function. Every week there was another CAT scan [a diagnostic imaging test] or treatment, and each time she'd talk to me, she would tell me about it and how she was slightly better or slightly worse. I couldn't take seeing and hearing about the treatments and what they were doing to her. I have such visual memories of certain times, like the time I took her to the beauty parlor. The stylist was combing her hair and every piece is coming out of her head. And I'm thinking to myself, nothing is working. This is it. I was so destroyed that my only means of survival was to try to separate a bit. We were holding on to each other for dear life. But part of me began to feel angry at her for putting me through this, and that is what finally helped me pull away.*

The involvement Lauren had with her mother both emotionally and practically for so many years left her depleted and depressed. She could not live her own life during her mother's sickness. "It's very important for a daughter to develop some effective boundaries and limits in terms of what she does for her mother, and to not put her own life on hold to the point that she risks neglecting her job, pushing away her husband, or even depriving her children of her attention and love," explains UCLA psychologist David Wellisch. "I found that daughters who don't put limits on their involvement with the illness are more prone to feeling depressed and angry over time. Whereas those who put limits on what they do are prone to feel positive about themselves," he says.

Lauren fell into the former group. Depressed and angry, she decided to get help and contacted a psychologist who works for Cancer Care, Inc., a cancer support organization based in New York. In therapy, Lauren began to see just how tied her identity was to her mother's and how she had relied so much on her mother to help her cope. Armed with this knowledge, Lauren began to disengage. First, she resisted the urge to call her mother as much, and although this meant speaking once or twice a day rather than five times a day, it was progress. But perhaps more significant, she stopped turning to Joan with her problems.

> *I turned to myself. I've developed a lot of inner strength through this. I don't lean on anyone anymore. I've learned to cope, to take one day at a time, to be happy. I didn't feel as if things were as urgent anymore, like she was going to die in two days and I had to be there to hear every little detail of her illness. I could get away from it, but my mother never could and that hurt a lot. Before my mother died, I said, "Mom, I know in the last year or so, I haven't always been there for you. Sometimes I've been a little selfish." And she said to me, "Lauren, don't ever feel that way. I love you no matter what."*

Joan also tried to let go of Lauren. She found other women with breast cancer whom she turned to for support and friendship so that Lauren could become a bit freer to focus on her own life and her own children. But once Lauren began to think of herself, she began to fear for herself.

> *The real thorn in my side is knowing that this can be inherited. I'm scared to death that I'll get breast cancer. I feel like my life has gone like my mother's life, and I feel like, why shouldn't I get it because I am her. I'm totally obsessive about this. I do breast self-exams every night and I unconsciously feel my breast while I'm walking down the street. I've woken up so many nights sweating, dreaming I was in the hospital on chemotherapy, dreaming I was losing my hair. I feel guilty because my thoughts should have been only about my mother, but I got riveted to myself.*

Her fears are not unusual. Many daughters believe that their mother's fate will be their own. The fact that there is a known hereditary factor in breast cancer risk has fanned the fears of daughters. Because they are like their mother physically, because they have the same hair color, the same hips, the same eyes, and maybe some similar personality traits, they think they have inherited everything from their mother, including a predisposition to breast cancer, explains psychologist Roberta Hufnagel. "But these other traits are not at all related to whether they're at risk for breast cancer," she says.

When Lauren's mother died in 1994, her own fears escalated. "My grieving turned into a fear of dying. I was very angry at everyone and feeling very lonely and scared," says Lauren. Whether it was a self-fulfilling prophecy or a mere coincidence, only six days after her mother died, Lauren found a lump in her own breast and felt certain that her own death was imminent. It turned out to be benign. A few years later, however, she had a similar scare, and all the images of her mother's death and all her fears came back to haunt her. Again, it was benign.

To help alleviate the fear, Lauren goes to a breast specialist every three months. Her husband, Jay, who stuck it out through those years when Lauren had pushed him away, is now her greatest support. Jay accompanies her on her doctor visits and stays on top of all the cancer research. "In a way, we made it through the worst of times," says Lauren. "We're both here to remember what happened and to deal with the future head on."

Lauren had considered joining the breast cancer prevention

trial, a large-scale study to determine whether the antiestrogen drug tamoxifen could prevent breast cancer in high-risk women. Lauren didn't qualify for the trial because she didn't have enough risk factors. She has even thought about taking the more radical path of prophylactic mastectomy, the procedure in which a woman's healthy breasts are removed preventively. "Honestly, I don't care about my breasts. When you watch someone you love so much, the person you're closest to in your whole life, go through so much pain for these breasts," says Lauren, gesturing toward her own chest, "you just don't want them anymore."

Recently, she decided to take the BRCA genetic test to see if she had inherited the gene mutation that increases a woman's risk of breast and ovarian cancer. Before she got tested, Lauren met with a genetic risk counselor, who calculated her risk of breast cancer and who talked to her about all the implications of the test, including her medical options if she tested positive. It's important for any woman who is considering this test to thoroughly understand the consequences for herself and her family (see *To Test or Not to Test*). Despite some of the drawbacks of testing, it was an easy decision for Lauren to make because she could not live with the uncertainty of not knowing. "I was ready to face whatever the outcome was. If it was positive, I was going to take my breasts off," she says. "There was no question in my mind." The test, fortunately, was negative, meaning that Lauren has probably not inherited the mutation. This brought her some relief. "It helped mentally. It's not a guarantee that I won't get breast cancer, but it released a little bit of my anxiety," says Lauren.

She was also relieved for her daughters, Rachel and Tori. "The hardest thing is to think about my daughters, because I can't bear for them to go through what I've endured. I'll never forget what I saw my mother go through. Every time there's some news about breast cancer, I sit in front of the TV and cry. I hope and pray that soon they'll come close to something so my girls don't have to suffer with this." Indeed, Lauren has made a concerted effort to make her girls independent. She saw it as a blessing that her second child was also a girl, so that the sisters would have each other to lean on if Lauren ever got cancer. "Rachel and

Tori are already best friends," says Lauren. "My mother used to say to me, 'I'll always be here for you.' I can't promise this to my daughters. Instead I say, 'Your sister will always be here for you.' The scariest part is looking at my girls and wondering who would take care of them."

But for Joan, who never dreamed that she'd have to break her promise to Lauren so early in her life, the end was filled with guilt and fear for her daughter. About four months before she passed away, she told Lauren about a dream she had. In the dream, Lauren was on a roller coaster. Her brother and his wife were in the back of the roller coaster, laughing, partying, and having fun. Lauren was in the front, sitting alone. She transformed into a little girl and reached out her arms and said, "Mommy, please come back. Mommy, I need you." Joan knew that she was her daughter's confidante and her support, and she worried about how Lauren would survive without her. "Well," says Lauren, "before she died, I said, 'Mom, I'm strong now. I'm going to be okay. I don't need you anymore.'"

It took Lauren about a year after her mother passed away, a year of just going through the motions of life, before she felt strong enough to return to the world without her other half.

FELICIA
EMORY, VIRGINIA

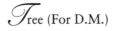ree (For D.M.)

From the stump of your breast,
green leaves are sprouting
with the certainty that birds
will nest again in this body
you celebrate daily
with a spirit of abandonment
only women like you can understand.

My mother's scar twists like a grapevine,
knotty and gnarled like the veins on her hands.

If I follow it to its source,
I see the flesh that formed me.
My mother, even without tattoo, is like you:
she gave up her breast, and she does not need it.
And I don't either anymore.

Felicia

When Felicia was young, her mother said, "When you're eighteen, you can get a nose job." Later on, when Felicia completed her PhD, she said, "You're not cut out to complete big projects." Recently, she said, "One reason I have breast cancer is because you kicked my breasts when you were little." Felicia's mother is not the June Cleaver type, not quite. On the other hand, her mother imbued Felicia's life with a cultural richness, a love of writing, art, music, and politics that has shaped her life.

Maybe this dichotomy led Felicia, a forty-three-year-old poet and professor of English at Emory and Henry College in Virginia, to say in our first interview, "My mother is my best friend." Perhaps she was hoping that if she said it, it would be true. Perhaps on that day she believed it. But later, after several phone conversations, e-mail correspondence, and much soul searching on her part, she corrected herself. "Although I have said that my mother is my best friend, she isn't. She's a puzzle, an enigma. I have dedicated much of my life to understanding who she is and why she is the way she is."

When Felicia's mother was diagnosed with breast cancer, it added an element of panic to Felicia's quest to understand her mother, a quest that occupies her thoughts and many of her poems. "To live with myself, I wanted to make sense of my mother and come to a reasonable relationship with her before she dies," says Felicia. Daughters who have not made peace with their mothers during their mothers' lifetime can suffer a great deal of guilt and regret after the mother's death. "The loss through death is so much more difficult when the daughter is left with unfinished business and bitterness," says psychologist Evelyn Bassoff.

Felicia's mother, though, is a survivor. She was diagnosed with advanced breast cancer seven years ago, when she was seventy, old by many people's standards but not by hers. She is an active gardener, an avid intellectual, an independent individual, and still has a firm hold on Felicia's psyche. It was a particularly horrifying diagnosis for the family, because twenty years earlier, Felicia's brother died of Hodgkin's disease, a cancer of the lymphatic system. Despite the bad prognosis, her mother has done surprisingly well. She had a mastectomy, followed by chemotherapy, which she had to stop for health reasons, and for five years she took the antiestrogen drug tamoxifen, a hormonal cancer therapy.

Prior to the cancer diagnosis, Felicia felt alternately cold and warm toward her mother. She dreaded the frank, judgmental, and sometimes brutal comments her mother would make about people. In contrast to her mother, Felicia appears meek, with her large glasses and her dark blond hair worn in a neat bob. She's quiet, extremely polite, and tries to be generous in her views of others. "My mother criticizes people for superficial things like their looks," says Felicia. "It took me years to wear glasses in front of her because she would cringe whenever I did. It took me years to outgrow the feeling that I was hideously ugly. I can only now say that I actually look *okay*." It's not that the two women have an outwardly hostile relationship. Though Felicia has been hurt, offended, and embarrassed by her mother, she has rarely confronted her. She has been so put off by her mother that on one occasion, she seriously considered cutting off all contact with her. Her father, a writer as well, who adores her mother, convinced her to try harder to understand her mother and not abandon her family.

When she feels warmly toward her mother, Felicia is thinking of her mother's admirable traits which have kept Felicia around this long. Her mother passed on to Felicia many of her passions, from her cultural pursuits to her talent for storytelling, a family tradition that influenced Felicia's decision to become a poet. She handed down her hobbies like gardening, a subject they often share stories about, and a love of baking. "When my mother got sick, in fact, I began making cakes in a rather obsessive way. I think it was a way of centering myself, but it was also a way of connecting to her, because she was a great baker. My childhood was filled with wonderful cakes and breads and pies," says Felicia. "I remember her yeast rolls, hot from the oven, full of butter—the best biscuits I ever had (I ate them with butter and grape jelly) and coming home to vanilla cake with homemade chocolate frosting or her peach pies." Felicia began writing down recipes (she and her mother both baked without recipes), and she published a small cookbook called *The Best 50 Bundt Cakes.*

Felicia has also written many poems about her mother, some that are sentimental and others that are, as she puts it, "unkind." "If I don't have regular contact with her, despite how much she may get on my nerves and no matter how much I have to put up with to try to be with her, I miss her and need her in certain ways," says Felicia. "So I have tried to hang in there, and I have spent much of my life working on a relationship with her to show I could have one and because I do feel a blood tie that I want to honor." At the same time, she has had to distance herself physically and emotionally from her mother and has built a shell against her mother's verbal insults. Before her mother got cancer, there were times when phone calls were brief and visits were infrequent. Once, she went two years without seeing her parents.

When her mother was diagnosed, Felicia fell into a deep depression, fearing that her mother would die. Her mother asked Felicia to take off work to go home to South Carolina the week before surgery was scheduled rather than afterwards. Her mother wanted to enjoy a visit with her daughter instead of having Felicia take care of her after the surgery. "We had a lot of fun together. We went to a movie and a Halloween party, and we were cheery, but after the surgery, I left and cried all the way home." Her sadness stayed with her for months.

"Whenever a mother becomes very sick, the daughter understandably can become overwhelmed with sadness, very frightened or very angry, because the mother-daughter relationship is by its very nature so intense," says Bassoff. A mother's dying is one of the worst things that happens to us in life. Felicia slept in her study for a month rather than with her husband, going off into her own world. She was worrying about the work on the relationship that still needed to be done. "I just wasn't ready for her to die," says Felicia. But her mother didn't die, and as soon as Felicia realized that there was still time, she began to let her mother in, little by little, through cracks in her hardened shell. Her mother's cancer, with the threat of death, created an opening, allowing Felicia to view her mother with sympathy, as a vulnerable human being.

> *With the breast cancer, I felt sorry for her and began to think it was totally unfair for her to go through it because she hasn't had the easiest life. She's had a lot of disappointments and it seemed very unfair for her to get sick after having to nurse her dying son. It was also hard to see her come out of it looking so frail when she had been such a vivacious woman. That made me realize I wanted to be cozier with her. I wanted to be there for her, to cheer her up, to make her feel like she had a wonderful life. I tried to be a more amenable daughter, someone who didn't disagree so much, who tried to be more accepting of her ways.*

Though her mother lived too far away for Felicia to help in the day-to-day caring (her mother is fiercely independent and didn't ask for help), she began to call and visit her mother more often. "It made me feel a deeper connection to her. The cancer made me stop hiding so much of myself from her," says Felicia. "Part of our not having an ideal relationship is just me being sort of distant. I was reading in a Jungian book by Kathie Carlson [*In Her Image: The Unhealed Daughter's Search for Her Mother*] that we are socialized to expect mothers to be stereotypical good mothers and disappointed when we get *mother* instead of *Mother*, because in reality we get human beings that are much more complicated. My longing for the stereotypical mother has perhaps been a factor in my poor relationship with my mother."

Felicia has begun to open up to her mother, not necessarily revealing deep emotions, but sharing her stories about her work, her own little boy, and her life. They also have spoken at length about her mother's treatments and her progress, a topic that typically generates a certain level of intimacy when shared. "When my brother got cancer, we didn't talk as much. It was such a shock. I felt left in the dark. This time around, we talked a lot. She told me some of the gritty details about her doctor visits, the medicine, the chemotherapy, and the side effects," says Felicia. Allowing a mother to speak about the details of the treatments and the side effects can relieve some of her anxiety surrounding them and can also make a daughter feel more involved with her mother's experience, which serves to relieve anxiety for her as well, says psychologist Roberta Hufnagel.

> *I see myself as a handmaiden to her, someone to help her enjoy the time she has rather than there being something in it for me. It sometimes comes at great emotional cost to me as I create a schism between who I really am and who she needs me to be. I'm a very independent, autonomous person and pretty much have run my own life since I was very young. But because she needs me, I have to abandon some of that autonomy or some of my beliefs about how things are. I have to turn a part of me off, and just be with her, just be there without questioning or assessing or judging or anything. I've become the person she can open up to and let her hair down with. It's wonderful that I can be that person, but it's sometimes hard for me.*

There is often a sublimation of one's self when a daughter has to be there for her mother, says Evelyn Bassoff. She might repress her needs, her feelings or thoughts, and this can be particularly difficult when a daughter is trying to emotionally separate from her mother, to individuate, which often happens in the teenage years and in young adulthood, but for many women, like Felicia, may not happen until even later in life.

> *I've always thought my quest was to understand her and know her, because then it would make more sense to me why she is the way she is. But part of why I'm hanging in there is because I'd like her to know me too. I don't know that she will ever know me. When she got cancer, I really did think she was going to die because she wasn't young and it was advanced, and the whole idea of her dying at that point really upset me a lot, because I'm not ready for my mother's death. I don't think we have peace yet, I don't think we know each other as well as I'd like.*

2

MOTHERING MOM

"Sometimes my mom would suffer in pain through the night because she didn't want to wake me up, and that would break my heart. I just wanted to be able to give her morphine when she needed it. I have the rest of my life to sleep."

Sunshine London, 24

SUNSHINE LONDON
LAS VEGAS, NEVADA

Sunshine London awoke at 5:30 in the morning and for a fleeting second, thought it was time to go surfing. It had been her routine, rising during the small hours of the day and heading off to the ocean to ride the waves. But now, she heard her mother's cries of pain and leapt out of bed to get the morphine. Only a few months ago, when Sunshine's father called to tell her that her mother's breast cancer had metastasized, the carefree life she was leading at the age of twenty-two came to an abrupt end.

That life was set in Santa Barbara, California, a place known for its dramatic natural beauty and year-round great weather. With her bleached blond hair, large brown eyes, and cheekbones the size of plums, Sunshine blended right into the Southern California scene. She lived thirty paces from the beach and divided her time between surfing, attending the University of

California at Santa Barbara, and modeling, which paid her tuition. It was after a morning of surfing, only a few days after she had finished her last final exam for her last semester at college, when her father called with the bad news. "I got off the phone with my dad and immediately started crying. I thought, this was my nightmare coming true. My mom is the most important person in my life. I couldn't think of anything except to go home." That afternoon, Sunshine got in her car and drove home to Las Vegas.

Her mother's prognosis was not good. The cancer had begun to spread. She had eighteen inoperable tumors on her lungs. Later, it would spread to other organs and to her brain. She was given about a year to live. Sunshine moved home, and while her father put in long hours at work—he hosts a local TV talk show and manages medical practices—she nursed her mother, Rebecca. Toward the end of her mother's life, it meant almost round-the-clock caregiving. It was the biggest responsibility she had ever taken on, and it was emotionally and physically exhausting.

Sunshine's typical day began with her mother's anguished wake-up call. Sunshine prepared the morphine, then rubbed her mother's back until the pain went away and her mother fell back asleep. She went downstairs and made her mother oatmeal and fruit or a smoothie for breakfast. She had many details to handle, such as organizing her mother's medications. "There were so many medications that she had to take every day. I had these little organizer boxes, divided into Monday through Friday, breakfast, lunch, afternoon, and dinner," says Sunshine. When her mother was awake, they sat in her bedroom and talked. "Sometimes I read to her, because she had detached retinas from the tumors behind her eyes and couldn't read anymore, and sometimes we watched soap operas together," she says. Sunshine massaged her mother's body and her feet to relax her, and she often had to cajole her mother into being a more cooperative patient. "It was frustrating because she would have two bites of food, and would not eat anymore, and I had to try to urge her to eat. She also fought me because she didn't want to wear her oxygen mask." Sunshine had some training in caring for patients—

she had taken a six-month medical assistant certification program—but while she was adept at the pragmatic details of caring for her mother, she was in no way prepared for the emotional anguish of the job. "It was very hard for me to see her in pain and deal with whatever symptoms cropped up each day, like a numb tongue or her toenails coming off. After I'd spend time with her, I used to go in my room and cry. I felt so helpless that I couldn't take the pain away, that I couldn't stop her from deteriorating," says Sunshine.

"It is extremely tough for daughters to assume the caregiving role because the mother-daughter relationship is set up in the other direction, where mothers from conception onward are the caregivers," explains Roberta Hufnagel. In a normal life history, daughters deal with this issue when their mothers are much older, but breast cancer often brings this into life before daughters are ready to take it on. "There can be a deep emotional trauma of having to reverse these roles, something many women aren't even aware of," adds Patricia Spicer, ACSW, breast cancer program coordinator for Cancer Care, Inc., a national support organization for people with cancer and for their families.

Sunshine had become her mother's caregiver, Rebecca's one-woman army warding off symptoms, pain, and discomfort, her outlet for conversation, her consoler, and her confidante. In the afternoon, while her mother slept, Sunshine cleaned the house, did the laundry, and prepared dinner. Any spare time she had, she tried to read up on all the treatments her mother was taking, and she became certified in Reiki, an alternative therapy for relieving pain. Every day Sunshine made one trip outside to get lunch for her and her mother and to run to the drugstore. Her mother usually needed some new drug to treat whatever medical crisis or uncomfortable side effect arose that day.

As difficult as it was for Sunshine to care for her mother, it was also gratifying and worthwhile. "When a mother and daughter are close, the illness can bring them back to something very basic, and that's the care of the body," says Evelyn Bassoff. She adds, "Many women have become close to their mothers because they took care of their mothers' bodies. It's a very powerful experience, the physical contact between mother's body and child's body, something that's lost during adolescence. Now there's a return to basic caregiving, like washing the mother's body."

Sunshine's caregiving, however, didn't begin and end with her mother. She had five younger siblings: three school-age sisters who were seven, ten, and twelve, and two teenage brothers. Although the boys could fend for themselves, the girls needed someone's help, and the only people available to help were Sunshine and her grandmother. Between the two of them, they had to give the girls their meals, get them ready for school, buy their supplies and clothes, and tend to their emotional health. "It was difficult because it was a lot to do and because I couldn't stand seeing my sisters so sad," says Sunshine.

For support, Sunshine had nowhere to turn except back to her mother. "When my mom cried, I wouldn't cry. I became this super-strong warrior person, who was comforting and happy. But sometimes when she was just hanging out in bed, I'd come in the room and start crying hysterically. I'd lay with her and we would just hold each other. I'd say, 'Mom, you can't die, you can't leave me.'" Every day Rebecca thanked her daughter for her help and companionship and told her that she knew what Sunshine was doing was arduous. "Just hearing how grateful she was made it all so much easier and worthwhile," says Sunshine.

What really helped her sanity was that Sunshine adored and admired her mother. Faced with her mother's deteriorating health, Sunshine felt an urgency to learn everything that she could from her mother, before it was too late. Rebecca had an impressive list of accomplishments. She was an English professor, studied art history, spoke French, and taught drama. Sunshine was also impressed by her personality. "She was such a high-spirited person. She literally never got grouchy," says Sunshine. As daughters, we typically look to our mothers for wisdom, even in times of life-threatening illness. "Even when the daughter takes care of the mother in a physical way, the mother still remains the daughter's teacher and guide. The mother is still a generation ahead of the daughter and still has lessons to impart," says Bassoff. "There are profound changes that can happen when you are really with somebody who is very ill."

"I was like a sponge. I asked her as many questions as I could because in the back of my mind I had a fear that she was

going to die soon," says Sunshine. "I asked her about past relationships, about sex, about my dad, about the children [her sib-
lings], how she felt about controversial issues, what her favorite
color was, the kinds of music she liked, and what she used to do
for fun before she got married." Sunshine sat by her bedside as
her mother regaled her with stories. After they talked for an hour
or so, Sunshine would make up some excuse to leave the room,
and she'd run downstairs and write everything in a journal. "The
whole time, I was thinking that my sisters aren't going to remember her. I always felt guilty because I had her during the time a
girl needs her mother the most—when you're changing into a
woman and have so many questions about life—and my sisters
wouldn't. I just wanted to write down every little thing that she
thought about so when my sisters got to that age, I could tell
them exactly what Mom thought on the subject."

Sunshine was also writing for herself. She was learning
about life through her mother's stories. Before her mother died,
Sunshine got a tattoo, an image of a vine of daisies climbing up
her forearm. "It represents growth. I thought I did more growing
in one year than I'd ever do again in my entire life. The vine is
there on my body reminding me of what I went through. People
forget. It's on my forearm so I don't."

As her mother got sicker, it became harder and harder to
talk to her. "My dad and I used to sit up late at night and say
how much we missed just talking to Mom," says Sunshine.
"Even though she was there physically, mentally she had changed
so much because of the morphine. She didn't know who we were
sometimes. She'd get confused and she'd say strange things and
act erratic." It also was difficult to see her mother go from a
curvy, robust woman to a frail, elderly looking one. "It was hard
seeing her try to walk, she had to go two inches at a time. She
was so skinny and tiny, I felt that if I touched her, she would fall
down," says Sunshine.

Sunshine struggled with many issues during the last stages
of her mother's life. One of the hardest was not having much
control over the decisions made about the course of her mother's
care. Her father was on a quest to save her mother's life, and like
many husbands of sick women, he coped with the situation by
doing intense research on the available treatments. He did not

want to give up and was willing to try anything, so he signed up his wife for various experimental treatments and sent her to a number of alternative centers, places in Mexico and as far away as Germany. "There were days that she'd be vomiting and he'd still want her to get on a plane and go," says Sunshine. "I didn't understand that from a medical point of view. I thought we should quit trying to fight this disease that's already won. I thought we should let her rest peacefully."

Sunshine and her parents are religious, but she says she felt her parents were accusing her of being unfaithful to God because she wasn't hopeful about her mother's outcome and because she wasn't proclaiming that God was healing her. "I couldn't help it. I studied biology and I knew what was happening to her cells, and I'd see all the MRI results [an imaging test used to view cancer] and I'd be with her when she was in pain all through the night," says Sunshine. Witnessing her mother suffer some excruciating moments had already put serious strains on her faith. There were a few times, as her mother's condition worsened, when Sunshine wished that it would all be over. "I would come into my room after being with her for hours, when she was in pain and crying, and she'd finally get to sleep, and I would ask God to please take her, I don't want to see her suffer anymore," says Sunshine.

She tried to stand up to her father, so they fought regularly during her mother's illness. "I understand why my dad did what he did. My dad was totally in love with her. He was totally supportive of her throughout the whole thing and my mom stayed so completely in love with him. It was just really hard for him to stop trying, and she just did whatever he suggested."

Rebecca passed away in October 1997.

I feel horrible saying this, but I had this feeling of relief inside. She was no longer suffering, and I was no longer suffering. I feel like I had the disease because I went through every step with her. I was with her through all the MRIs, when the doctors gave her more bad news, during all the chemotherapies, all the experimental drugs we tried, all the nausea and long nights of pain. I feel like I went through everything except the physical pain. It was horrible.

But I don't regret putting my life on hold one bit. I'm young and I have many more years to live. I gave a small portion of my life for a really big reason. But when it was over, I thought, I'd done nothing for myself for two years. I didn't have friends, I didn't go out, so I thought I was ready to go on with my life.

Unfortunately, her responsibilities didn't end with her mother's death. Sunshine had, with much trepidation, stepped fully into the parental role for all her siblings. Her father, in bereavement, had buried himself even deeper in his work and continued to keep long hours away from home. According to Sunshine, he was not emotionally available and was unable to console his children. "I'm their next of kin. They don't have anyone else to turn to. I knew that it was all going to come down on me when my mom died," says Sunshine, who still harbors some resentment toward her father for some of the decisions he made as her mother was dying and for not being there emotionally for her and her sisters.

The first few weeks after my mother passed away, my sisters slept in my bedroom on the floor. They were too scared to be alone. To get them to sleep by themselves, I had to go through the whole process with each of them of lying with them in their beds until they fell asleep. It took a few weeks. I also had to get their clothes together, take care of their needs, and cook for them. Cooking was one of the worst things I had to deal with, because I didn't know how to cook and all of a sudden I had to cook for six. I started out making a ton of mac and cheese, and spaghetti, then I progressed to tuna casseroles, chicken and rice, and I made a ton of salad. I used to break down and cry in the kitchen for no reason. Then before I knew it, it was December and I had to do Christmas. I was like a robot; I was still in shock and grieving for my mom, but I had to decorate the tree and buy the presents for five kids. It was a nightmare dealing with my dad with finances. I felt like a wife, because I was spending more than he'd budgeted and he was yelling at me. But I wanted to get them the best Christmas presents ever because my mom was gone and it was going to be hard enough. One night I was up until three in the morning wrapping gifts. After I went to sleep, I had a dream that my mom was wrapping presents with me. I was telling her how hard it has been without her. She told me I was doing a great job and she appreciated it. I had felt very unappreciated before that. I remember feeling better since I had that affirmation from her, even though it was just a dream.

Sunshine convinced her father to hire a nanny for the girls so that she could stop playing the role of mom and finally do something for herself. After Christmas, she packed up and moved to San Francisco, where she had enrolled in a fine arts graduate program, something her mother had encouraged her to do. But within hours of her arrival, one of her sisters called her, crying into the phone, and proceeded to call her every day. Sunshine felt homesick herself. "I just realized that it wasn't time for me to be away from home." So no sooner had she unpacked than she packed up to return home.

During her mother's illness, Sunshine rarely went out socially, but on one of those evenings that she gave herself a break, she met a guy, and they ended up dating, after much persistence on his part. Dating is an overstatement. They talked a lot on the phone, and the guy, Chris, visited Sunshine at home when she needed consolation or support. A few months after her mother died, Chris proposed to Sunshine, and the two moved into their own home. But as soon as Sunshine moved out, her sisters would page her in the middle of the night and beg her to come home. One by one, they'd come over to sleep, bringing their tears and grief with them. Chris, knowing how much Sunshine loved her little sisters, was understanding of their visits, which tapered off over time.

For almost a year after her mother's death, Sunshine struggled with her grief and the burden of her sisters. "I've had a really hard time accepting the reality that our family is completely different without my mom. I envisioned that it wouldn't change. But everything changed. Everything has fallen apart and it's not a beautiful family like it was before," says Sunshine. She has also struggled with the question of what to do next. "I was trying to move on, but it was hard. I wanted to put this experience to use to help others, but things were so difficult, my family was in turmoil, and I didn't know what I was going to do," says Sunshine.

Around the anniversary of her mother's death, Sunshine met a woman who is a chiropractor and who also wanted to help women with breast cancer and other illnesses. The two women decided to open a center in Las Vegas that they called the Wellness Institute of Nevada. It's a place where people can go for different types of alternative and complementary treatments—Reiki, massage therapy, physical therapy, nutrition counseling, and even beauty treatments. "When my mom was sick, we had to go to ten different places to get all the treatments, so I had always had this vision of opening a healing center, where people could come to relieve all their symptoms," says Sunshine, her voice suddenly coming to life with her old surfer-girl enthusiasm and cheerful disposition. "This is big. This is huge," she says.

JILL FRIEDWALD
PLAINVIEW, NEW YORK

*W*hen Sandy Friedwald, a fifty-two-year-old mother of two, heard the news that she had cancer, she was certain that the diagnosis meant she was dying. To anyone, the word *cancer* invariably evokes panic and fear of death, a gruesome one at that. For Sandy, the news seemed decidedly not in her favor. "My lymph nodes were the size of plums instead of raisins," recalls Sandy. "From what I knew about breast cancer, if it was in your lymph nodes, that was it, you were going to die." Aside from having malignant lymph nodes, which in fact does not mean you're on the brink of death, what really scared Sandy was that the doctors weren't sure where the cancer had originated because there was no evidence of any tumors in her breasts. She feared that the cancer was either lymphoma (cancer of her lymphatic system), lung cancer, or pancreatic cancer—all of which have a potentially worse prognosis. "I really thought this is it," says Sandy. "I started cleaning the house and getting my things in order. I remember thinking that, when I die, I don't want people to think I'm a slob, so I started throwing out everything."

Sandy's nineteen-year-old daughter, Jill, stared incredulously at her mother. "My mom was a lunatic when she was first diagnosed. It was total chaos," recalls Jill, whose cherubic face belies her assertive voice powered by a healthy New York accent. "She was saying, there's no point to fighting this if I'm going to die anyway. We had a huge fight. I was screaming, 'How can you do this? How can you not fight for your life? You have to do this for all the people who have already passed away,'" says Jill, referring to the many friends they've seen die of cancer (they live on Long Island, infamous for it's high incidence of breast cancer). "It was a scary moment, because there I was telling my own mother to fight for her life." Whether she realized it or not, Jill was also fighting for her own life, at least life the way she had known it up until that moment.

Things would never be the same for Jill whether her mother took a passive or aggressive attitude toward her cancer. Her mother was put on Adriamycin, a type of chemotherapy, for about four months in order to shrink her lymph nodes, a necessary measure before she could have a mastectomy. (The doctors were proceeding under the assumption that Sandy had breast cancer, though they were not certain.) Because Sandy didn't get a definite diagnosis of breast cancer until she went in for surgery when the surgeon biopsied a lymph node to determine the type of malignancy, the family endured a painfully long period of uncertainty. In contrast, many families who face cancer suffer the most anxiety and fear when they hear the initial diagnosis and then during the following days or weeks when they have to absorb a small medical library's worth of information to make life-and-death decisions about treatment. Once the treatment starts, though, families tend to feel a little calmer and take some solace in the fact that the ill person is being treated. But Jill's family remained stalled in their depression and fear. During that stressful time, Jill felt that she had to be the strong one in her family. "My mother was anxious and scared, and my father wasn't much better. I had to keep both my parents together," she says.

Before the surgery, her mother, who works from her home

making gift baskets, cards, and other party items, fell into a depression and took to her bed, worrying about the end of her life and being too afraid to live. "She thought she was so sick she couldn't do anything, even after the side effects of the chemotherapy wore off. She would lie in bed, crying. She was very emotional, very snappy, and very tense. No matter what we did, nothing made her feel better," says Jill.

> *So I became the mother. I took over the mother role. I started doing all the laundry, doing the food shopping, taking care of dinner, and making sure the house was neat. It needed to be done, so I did it. It was difficult for me to do because it's a lot of work, and it was difficult for me because of the reason for doing it.*

Stepping into the mother's traditional role, as Jill did, is extremely common among adolescent girls and young women whose mothers have cancer. Many not only do household chores but take care of younger siblings and their mother. "Our research of families with cancer found that compared to boys, girls were assuming and being handed many more responsibilities within the family," says University of Vermont's Bruce Compas. But it comes at a cost to their mental health. Compas found that 24 percent of adolescent girls whose mothers had cancer were diagnosed with anxiety or depression. This increase in their responsibilities, his studies show, was largely to blame. For children younger than Jill, it's even more stressful because they haven't developed the skills to cope with the caregiving role they've assumed, explains Compas.

"I was angry at the situation," says Jill. "I mean I understood, but I was still mad that I couldn't be a kid anymore. That's what happened. I didn't see my friends as much and I didn't go out." The situation also created an internal struggle for Jill. She was in her second year of college, with a growing sense of independence from her parents, but she was suddenly called back home. A natural part of a teenager's development is being away from home and involving herself more with friends. "But this experience pulls girls back into the family, and that is part of the difficulty for them," explains Compas. When Jill returned home to help her mother, she and her mother experienced an awkward adjustment period, a kind of power struggle, until Jill relinquished her hard-won independence.

When September rolled around, Jill did go back to college, while her mother, with the help of a psychologist at Cancer Care, began to adopt more of a fighting spirit. The therapist helped her deal with her fears but also gave her suggestions for dealing with her doctors, her treatment, and the day-to-day hassles of being this ill. Says Sandy, "Having a close relationship with Jill gave me so much more strength to go through the surgery, the chemo treatments, and everything else, because I want to see her married, I want to see her children. This is the best part of being a parent. I don't want to miss out on it." She also began to think of her position as a role model to her daughter. "When you're first diagnosed, you're in the throes of it, and you don't know what you're doing," says Sandy. "But after a while, I began to hope that I would set a good example for Jill. I wanted to show her that when something like this happens, you don't just crumble and fall, you take every option and every step that you can to do the best you can." What Sandy realized is that even in serious illness, mothers remain teachers to their daughters. "The daughter is always looking to the mother to learn how to cope with sickness," says psychologist Evelyn Bassoff. "And as a mother takes on this role, even if she doesn't feel courageous at first, she becomes courageous just in doing it."

Jill began coming home on weekends, giving up the perks of college life—the social scene, the extracurricular activities, and the independence. She also came home for her mother's mastectomy, which turned into a disaster when the surgeon nicked an artery and her mother came very close to dying. After the surgery, Sandy suffered pain that was not adequately medicated, and the near-fatal surgery was followed by a bad infection that left her bedridden for a couple of months. After the surgery, Jill stayed home for a week or so to take care of her mother. "I was sitting with her and talking with her, getting her food and whatever she needed, making sure she had her arm raised or she was wearing her oxygen mask, being like a nurse. The one thing I couldn't handle was dealing with the bandaging. It was too upsetting to see."

Jill also kept her distance when her mother started on her second round of chemotherapy.

> *For a while, I didn't want to come home. I didn't*
> *want to see her sick. I couldn't handle it, but I spoke to her*
> *every day on the phone. When I finally came home, she*
> *looked like a different person. She had no hair, she had*
> *puffy dark bags under her eyes, her skin was pale, and she*
> *had lost some weight. It was pretty frightening. Your*
> *mother's the one who takes care of you and is always well*
> *and here she is looking so ill. But I didn't cry. I was always*
> *a rock. I never cried in front of her. I never wanted her to*
> *see me upset because that would upset her more. When I*
> *went back to college, sometimes I'd just cry to myself in*
> *my room.*

The summer of 1998, Jill came home and took care of things around the house. Sandy was nearing the end of her chemotherapy and was often tired and irritable. "My mom got kind of nuts after each chemo treatment. She acted like a two-year-old, which pissed me off. She got cranky, lost control of herself, but then later she'd apologize," says Jill. One issue that particularly irritated Sandy was having to relinquish her motherly duties. "She would kind of be resentful that I had to do things that she would normally do, like cooking and food shopping. That would upset her. She told me that it hurts her that she can't be as good a mother as she normally was. She was like a super mom before this."

While her mother was struggling physically and emotionally, there really wasn't anyone Jill could turn to for support. In fact, everywhere she turned, she found more trouble. "My mother had breast cancer, my father was a wreck, my brother is estranged from the family because he's an alcoholic, and he disappeared completely when my mom got sick, and my grandmother was diagnosed with thyroid cancer. My boyfriend was also giving me problems on top of that. He was living with us, but he was going through a hard time, and instead of helping, he was another responsibility I had to take care of on top of everything else. I needed someone to take care of me. I remember my best friend saying to me, 'You don't always have to be the

strongest person in the world.' I said, 'Yes, I do.' I feel like I had
to be strong for everybody else to help the family get by."

Sandy finished her chemo treatments in August 1998 and
then began a round of radiation therapy, a procedure that uses
radiation to kill any lingering cancer cells. The time between the
diagnosis and the end of treatment was about a year and a half,
far too long for Jill to go on filling her mother's shoes and being
the emotional support for the family.

> *I got more and more frustrated that I couldn't be
> young and do things I used to do. But I also knew that
> I had to do it. There's no question of whether I wanted to
> do it. I did it because I knew I was the only one. But I kind
> of gave up my youth. I became a thirty-five-year-old
> woman rather than a teenager. I had all the responsibilities
> of an older woman with her own household. I had a lot of
> stress and gave up a lot of my freedom. I used to go out to
> dinner with my friends, go to the movies, or run to the
> mall. Suddenly, I had to always check to make sure some-
> one was there with my mom, to see if she needed
> something, or if there was a doctor's appointment I had to
> take her to. I had to become much more responsible and
> less self-centered."*

On a deeper level, her mother's cancer has made her fearful,
afraid for her mother's life and for her own. "Both my mother
and my grandmother had breast cancer at age fifty-two. So I'll
probably get it," says Jill, echoing the sentiments of many daughters. Her fear, though, has been manifested in a distressing way—
in the way she views her own breasts.

> *I don't really like my chest. I haven't liked my chest
> for a while. I think it's probably a defense mechanism. I
> know in the future I'm going to lose one or both of my
> breasts. I never really thought my breasts were great.
> They're not too big, they're not too small, I just don't like
> the shape of them. But I started to dislike my chest more
> after my mother got cancer. So it's definitely a defense
> mechanism. I've definitely had the thought, "Why should I
> think they're so great if I know I'm going to lose them*

eventually." They don't bring me a great deal of sexual pleasure either because I'm very self-conscious of them. It's probably not a healthy way to be, but I have to feel that way for right now.

The stress has also affected her physically. Before her mother got cancer, Jill had been diagnosed with irritable bowel syndrome, a gastrointestinal illness of the large intestine that is often exacerbated by stress. The symptoms became significantly worse throughout her mother's illness, bad enough that she now has to take medication to control it. Even as her mother was recovering, Jill started seeing a therapist with Cancer Care because the stress of caregiving had become overwhelming. "The therapist told me I should start being a twenty-year-old girl again. She said I should have fun and do what I want. For so long, I let my own needs drop to the floor, and everybody else's needs go way up on the list."

The first thing she did was break up with her boyfriend. She needed someone who was willing to put at least an equal amount into the relationship as she did and who could offer more support than he needed himself. She started calling her friends and tried to hang out with them more and planned a weekend getaway with a few girlfriends. She started creating more balance in her life between caregiving and caring for herself.

> *I was nervous at first about being away from home, but my parents knew I needed to go out and have fun. Now I have times that I call "Jill times," when I do exactly what I want to do. One day I went whale watching, which is something I would not ordinarily do. Sometimes it was just visiting friends, going to the mall and buying myself something, or getting my nails done, things that pampered me in small ways. Even just getting out of the house made me feel freer. It became a luxury.*

Her mother is doing well now. She finished radiation treatment in November 1998, the cancer is gone, and she's back to her old level of functioning. Jill is back at school for her junior year, she has a new boyfriend, and after she graduates, she is planning to go into occupational therapy. Things have lightened up for Jill, but her mother's illness has changed her. "I became much more serious. I'm not as happy and bubbly as I used to be. I often worry about my mother. But it's also brought me and my mother a lot closer." Adds her mother, "Breast cancer can be a gift in some ways because it makes you so much more focused on what's important than what's not. It makes your life so much more precious. Jill was incredible through this whole thing, and it's definitely made our relationship that much more profound. I think we grew a lot from sharing this kind of raw human emotion."

3

SISTERS STICKING TOGETHER

"We pulled together tighter than ever, to make sure my mom was taken care of and we got through this okay."

Suzanne Fiering, 36

SUZANNE AND LISA FIERING
BOSTON, MASSACHUSETTS

*S*uzanne and Lisa Fiering went arm in arm with their mother to every doctor's appointment and every treatment. The three of them joke about it now, how the doctors would run and hide when they saw the trio approach. They cut a formidable presence—Suzanne and her mother both large in stature, and Lisa a solid athletic type. "The two of us were sewn onto my mother on either side," says Suzanne, thirty-six, the older of the sisters. When their mother was diagnosed in October 1993, at fifty-eight years old, the sisters worried most that she would have to go through this alone.

It was, after all, only one year before, almost to the day, that their father died suddenly of a heart attack at the age of fifty-eight. Their father was a generous, charismatic professor at Harvard University, whose funeral was attended by more than 650 people, at least a dozen of whom said that he was their best friend. "We all worshipped my dad," says Suzanne. "He was the light of each of our lives. His death, for the three of us, was so devastating that we were only just starting to stand back up after getting punched in the stomach. My dad was one of those partners who would have been with my mom every moment, and because he was medically sophisticated, he would have helped with the decisions, so we felt his loss even more. I was terrified at the thought of my mother being alone with this."

Suzanne, who was thirty-one at the time, was the first to learn of her mother's diagnosis. She is, in an ironic twist of fate, an oncology social worker, and she was employed at the Deaconess Hospital in Boston, where her mother had gone a day earlier for a needle biopsy, a minor procedure in which cells are removed from a lump through a needle inserted into the breast under local anesthesia. The lump had been detected on her mother's routine annual mammogram. Suzanne asked one of her friends, a nurse in the oncology department, to look up the results of the biopsy in the computer, rather than waiting for the doctor to deliver the report the following day. "I was standing at the nurses' station and my friend pulled the report up on the computer, wrote it down, and handed me the piece of paper," recalls Suzanne. "I had spent the past day and a half completely convincing myself that it was going to be fine. I had not one doubt or uncertainty that it wasn't going to be malignant."

The note read: "Consistent with early stage adenocarcinoma of the breast." Given her profession, Suzanne knew her cancer terminology well, having been routinely called upon to explain results like these to her patients. "But I was looking at this slip of paper and asking my friend, 'What does that mean?' All my knowledge of cancer went right out the window, and I became this very fearful, terrified daughter who was not ready to think of the possibility of losing her second parent within a year. I wanted my friend to look at it and say, 'Oh no, this can't be right; there's been a terrible mistake.'"

It was malignant, but Suzanne had enough encouraging information—the lump was only two centimeters and it was early stage—to know in her gut that her mother would be okay. The five-year survival rate for early stage breast cancer is over 97 percent. "I didn't think she was going to die, but I dreaded the idea that because I am the one who knows about cancer and the stronger one in the family, I'd have to convince my mother and my sister that she was going to be okay, and I dreaded the idea that they wouldn't believe me no matter what I said, and would have to live with that uncertainty. I was worried that my mother was going to be lying in bed every night thinking this was going to kill her," says Suzanne. Explains psychologist Bruce Compas, when people hear the diagnosis of cancer, they just hear *cancer* and they think of death. They don't hear the encouraging part of the news. They can't absorb that, even when it's early stage cancer and very likely curable.

It was late in the afternoon when Suzanne left work and went to the gym, where she knew her younger sister, Lisa, would be working out. "I didn't want to tell her over the phone, because when my dad died last year, Lisa was out of town, in Arkansas, and it was a nightmare having to tell her over the phone, her having to be alone all night. It was awful and it really affected her," says Suzanne. On her way to the gym, she tried to plan the best way to deliver the news. She found her sister on a stationary bike and just blurted it out.

Lisa, who was twenty-eight, burst into tears. "I was just coming out of the numb phase from my father's death. I just couldn't believe that it was malignant. I just thought, this can't possibly happen to one family in the span of one year." She was incredulous, as many people are when they hear that cancer has invaded their family. But there wasn't much time to sit and cry over the information. The sisters still had to tell their mother. "This is not something children should have to do," says Lisa, "but we couldn't let the night go by without being with her and telling her." Suzanne knew enough about cancer to be able to inform her mother what the next steps would be so she wouldn't be suspended in a state of panic until they could talk to a doctor the next day. The sisters dried their eyes and tried to pull themselves together. "It was very important for me that Lisa and I appear to my mom to be strong so she would get the message that we were going to get her through this," says Suzanne.

Calm and collected, they went over to their mother's home and were standing in the kitchen when Suzanne told her mother that she called the lab and got the biopsy results. Their mother said "Oh" and looked up. "I think she really didn't expect it to be cancer," recalls Lisa. "When my sister said, 'It's malignant,' my mother's mouth literally dropped open, and she just looked very shocked."

An oncologist friend of Suzanne's looked at the mammogram the next day. Suzanne and Lisa also paid a visit to their father's best friend, a surgeon. Their father was a highly regarded scientist, a member of the board of directors at Beth Israel Hospital in Boston, and most of his friends were doctors, so the family was in good stead. "All my mom's physicians got two-page e-mails about my dad's contributions to the hospital, and the loyalty of the hospital to him, and that my mom needs to get special attention," says Suzanne. The chief result of that memo was that their mother got an extra dose of attentiveness from the staff, and she didn't have to wait the usual time to get appointments with specialists. "Everybody said her cancer was small and contained, they used the term *garden variety*, and said that we had hope for a very good prognosis," says Lisa. "I haven't been the most optimistic person since my father's death, but I think I just had to believe that this was true. I desperately wanted to believe them. The following weekend, we were having my father's unveiling [in Jewish tradition, a service is held at the grave site on the anniversary of a person's death]. The only way I could cope was to hope that it was curable."

Within a few days, her mother, accompanied by a small entourage—her daughters and a couple of her best friends—went to the hospital for a lumpectomy. "It was just a very scary time," says Lisa, her voice quivering from the memory. "I don't even know how you get up in the morning and do that, go into the hospital and wait for your mother to go through that surgery when she's your one parent left." Suzanne and Lisa sat in the waiting room for a few hours, trying to keep their spirits up. "We were laughing and trying to make jokes," says Suzanne. "We were joking about what kind of wig she would wear for my wedding, which was only five months away. There was not one time when we said, what if it's really bad. We completely believed that she'd be okay, that she'd have her tumor out, then have her chemo, her radiation, lose her hair, then she'd be fine."

After their mother came out of the recovery room, Suzanne went in to see her. "She wasn't awake yet and she looked completely still. It really freaked me out seeing her in that hospital bed, to the point that I thought I was going to be sick. I think all the fear and sadness and everything else that I had been guarding against really hit me in that moment. I also think I was so upset because I had seen my father in the emergency room after he died, and the position that he was lying in on the gurney was the same position she was in," says Suzanne. "So I went out of the room, pulled myself together, and came back in and sat next to the bed and stared at her until she woke up. It was like I was willing her awake."

The surgeon had removed twenty-four lymph nodes, which is more than the usual number removed, but he was being extra cautious. There was no sign of cancer in the nodes, but her mother decided on a newer, more aggressive treatment approach that was just beginning to be offered to women with early stage cancer. In addition to the standard six weeks of radiation, she opted for six months of chemotherapy. "We all had questions about whether this was overkill. I had this moment of selfishness because I was getting married next spring, and I thought, I don't want her to be bald at my wedding," says Suzanne. "Our family had needed something really happy after my father died, and this wedding had become something fun to think about and plan. I was worried that the chemotherapy was going to ruin it for her, and if she was unhappy, I'd be unhappy."

After the surgery, the daughters camped out at their mother's for a few days until she recuperated. When their mother began chemotherapy, Suzanne, Lisa, or one of their mother's friends would bring her in for the treatment. Lisa, a human resources manager, worked in the hospital where their mother was receiving the treatments, so she was able to stop by during the sessions. Then one daughter would go home with her afterwards. At times, their mother got very sick from the chemotherapy; she also had painful sunburnlike patches under her arms from the radiation, and she lost all of her hair. The hardest thing for both daughters to deal with was that their mother didn't have her husband to help her through the emotionally and physically painful aspects of cancer treatment. "Even though my sister and I stayed with her a lot during the worst parts of the chemotherapy and radiation, in the final analysis your partner is gone and you're doing this on your own," says Lisa. "I remember one time I had gone with her for a chemo treatment and was sitting there, holding her hand, watching the IV in the other arm, watching them put poison in her, thinking, God, enough. She and my father were partners for thirty-five years of their lives. One person can only take so much."

Their mother took it all like the proverbial trooper. Her own sister and her mother were breast cancer survivors, so she had good role models. "She didn't complain a lot, I think because she didn't want to add stress to either of our lives," says Lisa. "But it's a double-edged sword. You know that there's more pain than she's letting on, and you want to be there for her, but on the other hand, watching your mother be an emotional wreck isn't easy either."

Suzanne was even more keenly aware of the pain their mother was not owning up to. With her background in oncology, she had seen people survive cancer and seen people dying from it, so she knew the reality of both scenarios. She also knew, in intimate detail, the many ways in which breast cancer patients suffer. "Having sat with women who are going through something like this, where there's so much pain and grief and fear, having felt it from other women for years, I knew in my soul that my mother was going through that too," says Suzanne. In spite of her training, Suzanne had a hard time seeing her own mother so sick. She recalls a few times when her mother told her not to come over after a chemo treatment. "My mom said, 'I'm fine. I'm just sleeping.' When I looked back on it later, I was really mad at myself for not going over there, just to be there when she woke up," says Suzanne. "But I think the reason I didn't go was that part of me didn't want to see her sick and nauseous and weak. It was a visual image of her that I couldn't tolerate. I need my mother; if I don't see her sick, I can convince myself that she'll be fine," says Suzanne.

Lisa felt just as vulnerable, if not more. "In some ways, I lost both my parents for a while. My mother, who is typically very motherly, had a very full plate. For a year, we had been caring for her emotionally after my father's death, and now we had to care for her physically and emotionally. My sister is very good at that because she's a social worker. I'm the baby of the family, and I was always taken care of, so my role switched very drastically, without warning, without lessons. I was forced to be emotionally supportive of my mother in ways I shouldn't have had to be at that age." Daughters just don't expect to have to be there for their mothers in this way so early in life, and they don't expect their mothers *not* to be emotionally there for them, says Cancer Care's Patricia Spicer. You grow up assuming that your parents will usher you through most of your life.

Being single, Lisa lacked the kind of support she needed when she came home after a long day of taking care of her mother. It also made her more fearful of the worst-case scenario, that her mother would die and she'd be alone, without a family. "I had my moments that I thought the cancer was going to kill her, when I was sitting on my couch, out of control, crying and saying, 'I can't be an orphan; this can't be happening,'" says Lisa. "I had some very close friends who were trying to take care of me. But at the end of the day, I'd get into bed alone and would cry myself to sleep a lot. That's when the reality of being afraid hits you."

"I have a whole new heightened awareness of my mom's mortality," says Lisa. "I have a complete and utter fear of losing her whenever she has the most minor symptom or when she goes in for her mammogram. It's a fear that I didn't know before my father died. Unless you lose a parent, you don't understand that protectiveness you have for the other parent that's left."

The three women spent a lot of time worrying about each other and trying to protect each other. Suzanne, who had difficulty turning off her professional self, was always trying to figure out how to solve everyone's problems and make her sister and mother feel better. "I spent half my time worrying about my mother and half the time worrying about my sister and most of the time eating Twinkies and pints of Haagen Daz," she jokes. Lisa and her mother, who both lived alone, had begun to look after each other. "We speak every morning and we speak right before we go to sleep," says Lisa.

By March, when there were only a few more rounds of chemo left, her mother started to act like herself again, and the girls started to relax. "I really felt like it was behind us that October," says Suzanne. It was the first year their mother participated in Making Strides Against Breast Cancer, a six-mile walk to benefit the American Cancer Society. Her hair was just beginning to grow back in. "When she came over that finish line, that was when I really thought, this is unbelievable," says Suzanne. "She has always been out of shape, so for her to walk six miles on a good day was an accomplishment, but still having remnants of chemotherapy drugs in her and to get out there and do that, I thought it was a testament to her emotional strength and the fact that she was physically fine."

In October 1998, her mother, flanked by her daughters, crossed the finish line of the Making Strides walk for the fifth time, an achievement that also marks the five-year anniversary of her diagnosis, when the risk of recurrence drops significantly. This milestone signifies the point when mother and her daughters can begin to feel that breast cancer is a thing of their past. After the walk, Suzanne and Lisa celebrated with a luncheon for their mother and twenty of her friends. They toasted their mother for surviving cancer and for becoming a hard-working volunteer for the American Cancer Society, for turning her unfortunate situation into something meaningful. "We were so psyched to throw the luncheon for our mother, but it was also for us," says Suzanne. "It really felt like we were closing a chapter for all of us."

4

MY MOTHER,
MY SELF

"My husband said I was waiting for this for twenty-three years. When I was diagnosed, it was like a weight was lifted off my shoulders."

Kathie Praml, 46

KATHIE PRAML
SAN FRANCISCO, CALIFORNIA

"When I was young, I vowed that if I ever had a catastrophic illness, I wouldn't deal with my kids the way my mom did with me," says forty-six-year-old Kathie Praml, a mother of two. It was a promise she would be called upon to keep.

"When my mother died, I was twenty-two with a nine-month-old baby, and the way I found out was that I got a phone call from my dad saying that she had died. She had been in the hospital, dying, for a week, and nobody had called to tell me," says Kathie. Once Kathie was old enough to move out of the house, she usually heard about the course of her mother's breast cancer after the fact, after a surgery was completed and her mother was back home or after one experimental treatment or another had been attempted without success. Toward the end, when her mother's health took a sudden and dramatic turn for the worse, nobody told Kathie.

Kathie and her brother were protected from the truth. It wasn't that her parents were being cruel. They, like many parents, thought this was the best way to handle their children, to spare them from having to face and cope with bad news. Her mother firmly believed that Kathie's focus should be on her new marriage and her new baby, not on her mother's failing health. "My mother was in a great deal of pain for the last nine months. She was a strong woman and she refused to let anybody know that she was in pain or to see her that way. My father was simply in denial, believing that if you don't talk about something, it doesn't exist," says Kathie. Shielding children from the truth about a parent's illness was more common back in the 1970s, when her mother had breast cancer, though it's still quite prevalent today, particularly when the children are young. But in trying to protect children, parents can actually do more damage, no matter how young or old the children are, according to Evelyn Bassoff. When a parent withholds information, it's as if she's telling a daughter that she can't cope with the truth, which can become a self-fulfilling prophecy. Moreover, it doesn't allow a child to spend the last precious days, weeks, or months with her mother, to express regrets, to express love, to say whatever needs to be said, says Bassoff. "I was never given the opportunity to say good-bye," says Kathie, "There were things that I disliked about my mom, and we used to fight a lot, but I loved my mother, and I never got to say that to her."

Aside from minimizing the extent of her illness, her mother often used scare tactics when she did discuss the cancer in its earlier stages.

My mother didn't exactly handle things the best way. Instead of saying, "Would you like to see me with no breasts," my mother called me into the bedroom one day and said, "Here, look," and lifted up her shirt with a flourish. Back then they did a radical mastectomy, so her breast was removed, her pectoral muscles were removed, and she was concave on one side. It was pretty scary. Then she did the same thing with her hair. She had been wearing a wig when her hair started to fall out, and then one day she suddenly ripped it off and she was bald. I can understand why

*she didn't want to wear the wig, but the way she took it off
made me afraid more than anything.*

There was another unforgettable incident that frightened
Kathie for life, though it wasn't something her mother orches-
trated. Three years after her mother was initially diagnosed, her
cancer metastasized. On a visit home, Kathie was asked to take
her mother to the hospital for a doctor's appointment. "I was in
the waiting room, rocking my own daughter in her stroller, and
sitting next to me was a woman who had a face mask on.
Suddenly it fell off, and she must have had cancer of the mouth
or nose because half her face was an open wound. It scared the
living daylights out of me. After that, I used to pray, 'Dear Lord,
if I'm to get cancer, please make it anywhere but on my face.'"
These frightening scenarios along with her mother's sudden
death made Kathie terrified of getting cancer.

> *I was paranoid. Any time I got sick, I thought it was
> cancer. If I had a hangnail, it was cancer of the hangnail. A
> cold was leukemia, a sore bone or muscle was bone cancer,
> a headache that lasted too long, a brain tumor. Because I
> had stomach problems, I thought I was going to be the
> youngest living stomach cancer woman in the world. And
> I exacerbated the problem by reading too much. I'd get out
> my many medical books, read about a disease and about
> the statistics, and think that I was going to be one of the 2
> percent that got it at my age. I had a doctor who was very
> good and understanding, but I think I paid for his new car
> with all my visits. He should have sent me to a shrink. The
> symptoms started appearing shortly after my mother's
> death in 1974 and continued until about 1985. I would get
> myself so sick with worry that I would throw up. I was
> hospitalized for it once because I couldn't stop vomiting
> and I lost fifteen pounds in eight days. At that time, my
> girls were three and five. It wasn't constant. I'd be fine for
> some time and then—bam, it would hit. I also had panic
> attacks, which usually occurred in the middle of the night
> and were set off by an everyday illness, like the flu or bron-
> chitis. I'd wake up sweating, my heart pounding, sick to
> my stomach, and feeling doom was near.*

For many daughters, their fear of cancer is set off by the trauma of seeing their mothers suffer horrible and painful deaths, says psychologist and cancer survivor Roberta Hufnagel. Once that image of mother crying in pain or mother vomiting or mother too frail to lift an arm is ingrained in their minds, it's extremely tough to imagine cancer playing out in any other less horrific way. Studies have found that some women who have this experience suffer from posttraumatic stress. It's irrational for most daughters to think that they will meet the same death as their mothers, as many daughters do realize, because the majority of women do survive cancer and the quality of life of patients has improved, but those disturbing images of mother are dogged and difficult to shake.

For many years, Kathie lived with her psychosomatic symptoms, which plagued her but also had become comforting, like any habit or pattern in life. Then her life began to change. Her husband's job was transferred from San Diego, where they lived, to San Francisco, and for two years he was commuting home for the weekends. "I suddenly became the mother and the father of two girls. There was nobody to cover for me when I got sick. I couldn't afford to be sick," says Kathie. She was also going to school part time and realized that her life was too full to be held back by a phobia. She finally went to see a psychologist who gave her an anti-anxiety drug, which she took on and off for several years. When she finally packed up her girls and moved to San Francisco, she vowed that it was all going to stop.

> I just began to think, I can handle things; it wasn't right to be so phobic and I didn't need to be. My symptoms started getting better when I'd tell myself they were an emotional response to not being able to say good-bye to my mother, to not knowing what was going on with her. I also did a lot of research and realized that there were so many strides being made in the treatment of breast cancer, between early detection and better chemotherapy, and I began to relax about it.

Kathie works as a costume designer for a community theater in San Francisco; she's an actor and a singer, a dramatic type who speaks passionately and is quick to find humor in even the traumatic stories she has lived through. As she let go of her cancer phobia, she became more lighthearted and began to enjoy life more. "In hindsight, it was a real waste of time and a waste of some very precious energy and good times I could have had with my children and my husband. I guess I always knew I was going to get cancer, but when I finally accepted that and stopped fearing that I'd die of it, I was able to live life more normally," says Kathie.

In 1997, at the age of forty-four, the age at which her mother died, Kathie herself was diagnosed with breast cancer. "My husband said I was waiting for this for twenty-three years. When I was diagnosed, it was like a weight was lifted off my shoulders. The hardest thing for me was not knowing. Waiting for the mammogram results every year was much worse than being told I had breast cancer. Now that it's here, I can deal with it. Once I knew it was there, I knew I had a job to do, and I could take care of it."

Because of her vigilance, the cancer was detected early. The tumor was one and one-half centimeters, so she decided to have a lumpectomy rather than a mastectomy. Choosing the less aggressive of the two procedures shows, at least symbolically, how far Kathie had moved away from her phobia. "I always have felt that having my breast removed wasn't something I'd do unless I had to. My mother had both removed, and it didn't do any good, so what's the point?"

Kathie had seventeen malignant lymph nodes, which meant that her cancer was an aggressive type, even though the tumor in her breast was small, so she had chemotherapy and radiation, followed in February 1998 by the grueling stem cell transplant. In this aggressive procedure, a patient receives megadoses of chemotherapy, but before the chemo is administered, some of the stem cells, the seeds of all white and red blood cells and the foundation of the body's immune system, are removed and frozen. These stem cells develop in the bone marrow and would otherwise be destroyed by the high-dose chemotherapy. A woman is prepped for about a week to increase the number of stem cells, and then cells are harvested through her blood. After she receives several doses of chemotherapy over a period of three to eight days, the stem cells are returned to her body. For about a month, as these healthy cells are multiplying, her immune system is dangerously compromised, and she has to remain in isolation to avoid infection.

But given the trauma to her body, Kathie did extremely well through all the treatments. "I was one of the first patients at the cancer center who had absolutely zero side effects after the stem cell transplant," she boasts. Typically, the symptoms are more severe than those for standard chemotherapy. Kathie is through with her treatments, and she has no sign of cancer. The combination of treatments, however, did eventually destroy her thyroid gland, so she needs to take thyroid drugs and her speech is sluggish. Psychologically, she took the cancer treatments in stride.

After all those years of phobia, of psychosomatic illness, of unnecessary doctor's visits, Kathie was uncharacteristically fearless when she was actually diagnosed.

> *I've never been depressed about the cancer. I've never thought of this as the end of my world or as a catastrophe. Some women quit living. I'm trying to show my kids that that's not what you have to do, that you have to live more, not less. So I've dealt with the whole thing with positive thinking and humor, which is how I deal with most things in my life.*

Kathie's younger daughter, Carly, who is twenty-one years old, was confused and somewhat angry about the way her mother dealt with the cancer. "Carly couldn't understand why my husband and I weren't sitting around crying about this. She asked, 'Why aren't you upset about something that can kill you?'" Kathie's answer was that for her, it wasn't the way to deal with the disease. Yes, she does feel certain that she will die of cancer, that cancer will get her before anything else, like heart disease or being hit by a bus, but she doesn't feel that she's going to die tomorrow or in the near future.

> *I've met a lot of people who think I'm very strong and some kind of hero because of the way I deal with it. It's just who I am. I think I do better in stressful situations than in calm ones. My voice of reason takes over. I don't*

see the point of wallowing in "Why me?" I've really changed since I was diagnosed, and much for the better. My relationship with my husband is 100 percent better than it was, because, it's a cliché, but I don't sweat the small stuff; there's no point in wasting that time.

One of the hardest aspects of the cancer experience for Kathie was having to tell her father. "Sometimes I feel that he is still mourning my mother's death twenty-four years ago. And he's been remarried longer to my stepmother than he was married to my mother," says Kathie. "It was a phone call I didn't want to make. I was worried that I'd hear all this wailing over the phone when I told him. I didn't want to be the one to bring him so much pain. I called him and said to sit down, and then I told him. Sure enough, he dropped the phone and started wailing. He's only lived with cancer *death,* first his mother-in-law and then his wife, and he didn't know that cancer *living* existed."

The phone call to her father as well as the calls to other family members and friends became an emotional drain on Kathie, so she decided to write a newsletter, which became an amalgam of humor, graphic medical details about her treatments, and updates on other areas of her life. She called it the Boob News and sent it to family and friends by e-mail. "I realized that people don't know how to react when you break the news to them. Some of them are silent, some say the wrong thing. I figured if they read it first, they could assimilate the information, then talk to me when they were ready to talk. I needed my closest friends and family to adopt my attitude, not their attitude. It's important for me not to have a lot of weepy criers around me now." Kathie also posted the newsletter on a breast cancer support bulletin board on the Internet, hoping to show women that they can be honest about what they're experiencing and still keep a sense of humor. Kathie's attitude has made it easier for her own daughters to handle. Says her older daughter, Stacey, who is twenty-four and living in Portland, Oregon, "I think the main thing that has affected my attitude is that my mom has always been upbeat when she talks to me, and she has never made us feel like it was this horrible thing."

Coming full circle, Kathie ended up coping with cancer much as her mother had coped, with an inner strength that allowed her to live her life without obsessing about the cancer and without being a burden on anyone. "I didn't ask my daughters to help me or care for me. I didn't really need their help, because I'm a strong person and my husband has been a great, great help," says Kathie. "My daughter in Portland asked if she should come home for my stem cell transplant. I said 'There's really no point; I'm just lying here feeling very bored.'" She did, however, live up to her promise to not keep her own children in the dark if she got ill. She has told her daughters everything from the beginning. Indeed, when they received the latest installments of the Boob News, written in full graphic splendor, they probably had more than enough details. Kathie e-mailed or spoke to her daughters every day during her treatments so that they were aware of her progress and prognosis. She didn't want there to be any surprises. If Kathie's health did take a turn for the worse, there would be enough time for her daughters to come and be with her, and for mother and daughters to say what needed to be said.

5

ADOLESCENT ANGST

"My breasts were growing, and at the same time I was worried about getting them removed or losing them."

Julie Alexander, 35

STACEY BUTLER*
WANTAGH, NEW YORK

*W*hen the women in the Butler family get upset, a bright pink rash spreads across their chests and necks. It's a hereditary thing. So when seventeen-year-old Stacey Butler of Long Island, New York, walked into her kitchen and found a huddle of red-necked aunts and cousins, she knew something was horribly wrong. The cause of this flush, she quickly learned, was that Stacey's mother, Ellen, fifty-seven, had breast cancer.

The women, a tight-knit clan, were reeling from the news, and while Stacey was trying to process the information as her own neck was turning crimson, one aunt turned to her and said, "You better behave this time and not act out, or you're gonna wind up killing your mother." That comment would certainly make the top ten list of the worst things to say to the daughter of a newly diagnosed woman. The aunt, brimming with fear and anger, had aimed her breast cancer rage at Stacey, and it was a reflex that had damaging consequences. "I could have killed her," recalls Stacey, her slate-blue eyes filling with anger just thinking

*Name changed.

about it. "For her to say that I was going to kill my mother was completely inappropriate. I still don't like her to this day." Her other aunts tried to defuse the comment, but Stacey, who suddenly found herself being catapulted past the stages of shock, sadness, and grief and landing smack in a pile of rage, exited the kitchen, raced passed the piano covered with family photographs, and retreated to her bedroom, alone and lonely.

The truth is, the aunt's accusation wasn't out of the blue. Stacey was not particularly well behaved and had certainly made life difficult for her mother. It's not that she was rude, a smart ass, or malicious. She just had a particularly bad case of adolescent angst that had been triggered, in part, by her broken-family status. Even now, carrying very little weight on her small frame and wearing her brown hair just to the nape of her neck, Stacey, twenty-one, looks like she's sixteen. She's usually shy and taciturn, and feels awkward revealing her feelings. Her parents had divorced when she was five years old and her older sister was eight years old. Her father was "a nasty alcoholic," according to Stacey.

Her problems began long before her mother was diagnosed with breast cancer. Stacey had a hard time in high school, not with the work as much as with her attendance. "I was always very sensitive, and I felt very shy and uncomfortable in school, so I started not going," says Stacey. The mother-daughter battles that ensued were frequent and furious, which explains to some degree her aunt's barb. Stacey, though, had recently transferred to a smaller alternative learning school, with the idea that the personalized attention would suit her better. That move, however, never got a fair test, because her mother was soon diagnosed with breast cancer, and Stacey had not yet established the solid foundation to handle it.

> It was scary for me and my sister because my mother has been the only parent we ever really had, and we didn't know if she was going to get better or if she was going to die from this. My sister was a nursing student and knew more about the clinical side. She takes things very hard, but she never lets it show. I had a lot of self-pity. I started going to school less because I couldn't focus on anything. I

went out at night and stayed up too late to wake up early enough to make it to school. I stopped going altogether for a few weeks. Also, some of my friends were in an alternative band, so if they did a show out of state, I just tagged along. I spent a lot of time with them and not that much time at home. I also started getting more into drugs. When I went out with friends, we would hang out at each other's houses, in parking lots or in the woods, and we almost always smoked pot. I also started doing harder drugs, often using before school or during lunch.

Behaving with more than the average level of adolescent rebelliousness is common among kids who are having difficulty coping with their mothers' illness. "Teenagers can become irritable; they can shut down emotionally or take up self-destructive behaviors, like using drugs, missing school, or driving recklessly," says Frances Marcus Lewis, RN, PhD, professor of nursing and health promotion at the University of Washington, and a leading researcher of children with sick parents. Often children and adolescents don't yet feel comfortable expressing their fear, anger, and other feelings, and often they have no one to talk to, so they work out their emotions through these behaviors. For an adolescent girl, a mother's breast cancer can also coincide, if not collide, with her own psychological development. The cancer disrupts her normal process of separating from the family and spending more time with friends, because the daughter feels that she's needed at home. The pull can be so strong, in fact, that some teens postpone their individuation from their parents during a mother's illness. But those who continue to separate and spend even more time with peers, as Stacey did, often end up feeling guilty, explains Lewis.

"I felt bad that I wasn't home when my mom was sick, but it was easier for me not to be here," says Stacey. "I had a lot of trouble seeing her sick and going to visit her in the hospital after her surgery." Because Stacey's father left the family when she was young, Stacey had always felt overprotective of her mother, as if her mother's good health was critical to her own well-being. She worried when her mother caught a cold, when she cut herself, when she was treated poorly by a romantic partner, or when she received any other insult of everyday life. So seeing her mother felled by a disease of this magnitude was like watching her lifeline slip through her fingers. "When a mother is ill, adolescents worry about their own future, they worry about who is going to take care of them if mom doesn't live, and they worry about their life plan going astray and the family falling apart," says Lewis.

> *The hardest thing for me wasn't the diagnosis; it was watching my mom get sick and not being able to do anything to stop it; it was watching everything that happens after the diagnosis, seeing her in the hospital after surgery, seeing her with the chemotherapy, so helpless for so long, watching her get worse and worse, and then slowly recover. She was tired and sick most of the time, and she hated being nauseous. She was miserable. She has always hated throwing up, so she would cry whenever she did. She had always been healthy, so for her to be sick for so long was horrible for her. She also hated the fact that she had to lose a part of her body. That scared me too. She felt like a man wasn't going to want her after she has these scars. She was just as upset about losing her hair. She had very thin hair to start with, so to lose what she had, she was very unhappy about it.*
>
> *There were good days when I'd be the good daughter and help out. But it was really hard for me. Once I picked her up at the hospital where she was getting the chemo. Her treatment wasn't done yet, and she was sitting there with no hair, with this needle in her arm. As much as I tried to push it away, seeing her there in the hospital made me face what was happening.*

Stacey was not able to face her mother or her fears, so she hid from them through her rebelliousness, wrapping herself in her self-destructive behaviors that had already become so comfortable to her. For that, she and her mother suffered. Even through the chemotherapy, Ellen was fighting with her daughter, trying to get her to go to school, to come home at night at a reasonable hour, and to stop doing drugs. Her mother, under the oppressive influence of chemotherapy, was tired, irritable, and often depressed, which intensified the fighting. Tempers were raw. "There were days when I fought every word she said," recalls Stacey. "She was so uptight and not feeling well, and I was making her anxious on top of that." Stacey and her older sister would also get into fights, as many sisters do. "But there was so much anger and rage in the house that all the little things built up, so that a fight over borrowing a shirt would end up with us screaming at each other," says Stacey.

Nothing was normal. Not even the much anticipated coming-of-age ritual of learning to drive. The experience made her mother so nervous that a driving lesson would inevitably end in a shouting match between them. One time, Stacey, enraged, simply got out of the car and walked home.

Things came to a head when Stacey started coming home high on drugs. Ellen had kicked her husband out of the house after twenty-five years of marriage because he was an alcoholic. It took everything she had to come to that decision, and when she did, she had no tolerance for alcohol or drug abusers in her house. "My mom gave me the choice to quit drugs or leave. It was a tough-love thing. I tried going into a rehab program for a few days, but it was too restricting and I stopped going. So I left home and moved in with my dad for a while. I think my mom did the right thing. It wasn't fair of me to put her through my problems when she was going through so much as it was."

The move was hard on Stacey because she felt no emotional connection to her father and, quite the opposite, disliked him immensely. She also had to endure his dismal lifestyle. "My father was still drinking. He lived in a single-room-occupancy building, so he had one room that we shared, and we had to share a bathroom with everyone else on the floor. The place was roach-infested, had mice, and had a pervading odor of cat litter. We lived on his social security check and had to eat in soup kitchens. It was a nightmare."

Aside from being miserable in these squalid conditions, Stacey missed her mother. She missed all the stimulating conversations they'd have and her mother's constant caring and concern, which earlier had felt like nagging. Stacey started attending school again and gradually stopped using drugs, mostly, she says, because she grew out of the phase. She was allowed to return home and in the fall, enrolled in a junior college where she studied psychology, doing well enough to make it onto the dean's list. "By then I had become a little more responsible, so things were better with my mom. I was really subdued because I had to leave the house, so when I came back, I was behaving a lot better," says Stacey. Her mother, meanwhile, had finished her chemotherapy and had more energy and less anxiety. The worst of things—Stacey's rebelliousness, the fighting, and Ellen's cancer and treatments—have faded into their past. But it's hard to feel that cancer is ever behind you. Ellen often gets depressed wondering whether the cancer will come back. Stacey feels deep sadness for her mother, especially during the times when her mother is feeling down. Mother and daughter have grown much closer; however, Stacey still can't talk to her mother about the days when she had cancer. Anything but that. It's still too painful a topic to broach.

KELLY JACKSON*
NEW BRUNSWICK, CANADA

When Kelly Jackson's father came home one crisp April morning in 1975, he went through his usual ritual, taking off his hat and coat, unknotting his tie, and slipping off his overshoes. Then he stopped and looked at eleven-year-old Kelly and her older sister, who were standing in the hallway, and said, "Your mother has cancer." He walked right past them and went into the kitchen, closed the door behind him, and began to cry. The next morning, Kelly got up to get ready for school, went downstairs, and found her father still sitting in the kitchen. He had cried all night, already mourning his wife's death, believing that a diagnosis of cancer led to one's immediate demise.

Kelly's mother didn't die. Today, she is a twenty-three-year survivor and in great health. After she was diagnosed, she had a mastectomy and appeared to be cancer free, until a lump was found in her other breast a year later. She had another mastectomy, received radiation therapy, and then her doctors put her

*Name changed.

on a strict maintenance program in which she went for tests every three months for five years. The doctors told the family that survival rates go down when cancer goes from one breast to the next, so for the next five years, Kelly's family was always on edge. "We used to hold our breath after she went in until we'd get the phone call a week later to let us know whether it was back or not. I spent the last part of elementary school, junior high, and high school going through that every three months, holding my breath," says Kelly, who lives in New Brunswick, Canada.

> *When my mom first got breast cancer and was in the hospital, my dad kept me out of school for a couple of weeks because he said I was crying too much and he didn't want me to go to school in that shape. I understand why he did it, but if I had gone to school, I might have been able to keep my mind off it. At home, I just cried most of the time, and when I wasn't crying, I was really moping. I remember that as being two years of Hell. It was really hard, too, because I had no one to talk to. Because my parents were older than most of my friends' parents, I had no friends who were going through anything at all similar.*

Nor could Kelly talk to her parents or her three sisters about her fears of her mother dying. "We knew we weren't supposed to mention what had happened to Mom. The feeling was, don't mention it because we don't want to tempt fate about it happening again." This left Kelly to worry and wonder alone. Not talking about cancer to children is one of the most damaging mistakes a parent can make. According to a study by Frances Marcus Lewis of the University of Washington School of Nursing, children who are between the ages of eight and twelve when their mothers are diagnosed with breast cancer fear that their mother will die from the illness. But many parents don't recognize their child's fears, or they dismiss them with a "Don't worry, sweetie," rather than a real heart-to-heart conversation. "Mothers try to protect the child and in so doing push the child away at the very time when the child is afraid of losing Mommy and would benefit from some kind of connection," says Lewis.

Kelly's mother was emotionally unavailable, so little Kelly naturally gravitated to her father. "It drove me closer to Dad, because you don't want to be close to someone who's just going to be leaving you," says Kelly. It's hard to be close to someone who, you feel, is already pushing you away, as Kelly's mother was unintentionally doing. But Kelly couldn't really talk to her father either, so she was left to deal with her fears about her mother's cancer on her own.

Her fears festered and multiplied like a malignancy, culminating in a fear of becoming a woman. "When I hit puberty, I remember thinking that Mum had breasts and she had to have them removed and that was going to happen to me too when I got breasts. I went from not knowing anything about cancer and breasts to thinking this disease happens to every woman. That was really scary." Witnessing her mother become sick and disfigured because of her breasts introduced Kelly to the notion that her body, her woman's body, can betray her. Daughters learn about their own sexuality, their identification as women, and their feelings about their bodies largely through their mothers. "Some teenagers whose mothers have breast cancer show a reluctance to reach that stage of development where one starts to become a woman, to develop breasts, and therefore possibly to become the target for breast cancer," says Margaret Burke, SCW, social work supervisor at Cancer Care in New York.

> *I didn't want boobs, plain and simple. They were for everybody else, but I didn't need them. I didn't want them, but I got them anyway, and they kept growing. They grew to be extremely big. I would deliberately buy bras that were too small, as a way of denying how big they were. You couldn't get me to dress like a female either. I was very much into pants and things that looked more masculine. A lot of big sweat shirts. I was hiding my body. I remember that I was only fourteen when I considered having surgery to get them made smaller or nonexistent.*

Because her mother survived breast cancer, Kelly was able to moderate her fears about her own risk of cancer. That is, until Kelly's older sister, who was forty-eight years old, was diagnosed

last year with advanced breast cancer. By the time she was prop-
erly diagnosed, the cancer had already metastasized to her bones
and her lungs, and there was little that could be done to save her.
She died only five months later. Her sister's doctors weren't pay-
ing enough attention to her symptoms, and Kelly blames her sister's death on the poor health care in the rural community in
Canada where her sister lived. But despite these rationales, Kelly
was again in a state of panic.

> *I was in utter disbelief because she was the one sister
> I was closest to. She was also the one who was into eating
> healthier foods, she always took vitamins, took care of
> herself as much as possible, and was the only one in the
> family who has never had a weight problem. I thought if it
> could happen to her, none of us are safe from breast can-
> cer. It blew me away and it blew my husband away, too.
> We both felt the very real possibility that this can happen
> to me, too. I got pretty freaked out about my own risk. I
> don't walk around every day worrying about it, but I can't
> take a shower without thinking about it and checking for
> lumps. I'm always checking to make sure that nothing's
> changed. If anything changes at all, I go into full panic
> mode. I think, it happened to my sister and I am next.*

Coincidentally, a month before her sister was diagnosed,
Kelly finally went for the breast reduction surgery she had been
thinking about for more than fifteen years. She happily went
from a size EE cup to a C. She would have had the surgery sooner, but she says people made her feel vain. She made the decision
partly because she felt self-consciously big and partly because the
weight of her breasts made her feel uncomfortable. She had a sore
back, she had grooves in her shoulders from the bra straps, and
she had bad posture. But she was also swayed by breastcancer.

> *I couldn't do a breast self-exam adequately. You can't
> find your way through that much breast tissue. I was get-
> ting to the point that every month I was noticing fibrous
> cysts. I was going to have to start keeping a scorecard, just
> to keep track of what I had where. That's not the kind of
> thing you want to write down in your diary. My doctor*

agreed that with my family history, having a reduction might lower the risk of a lump going undetected for a long period of time. It wouldn't lower the risk of something developing, but it would increase my chances of finding it sooner. When my sister was diagnosed a month later, I knew I had made the right decision. I have absolutely no regrets about reducing my breasts. I always disliked them anyway.

JULIE ALEXANDER
REDONDO BEACH, CALIFORNIA

*L*ate one night after attending a party at Hunter College in New York City, Julie Alexander, then a nineteen-year-old sophomore with hazel eyes and long blond hair, was on her way back to her dorm room when she passed out a few yards from her door. She hadn't eaten anything but a few carrots and celery stalks for a week. When she came to, she tried to crawl to her door. "I didn't know if I could even make it. I thought I was dying. It took everything I had to get into my room and get onto the couch, where I fell asleep. That really scared me and that's when I decided to see a therapist," says Julie, who is now thirty-five and living in Redondo Beach, California.

That night marked the nadir of her eating disorder that began six years earlier, in 1976, in Cherry Hill, New Jersey, when Julie was only thirteen years old and, not coincidentally, when her favorite aunt, Flossie, was diagnosed with breast cancer. Her aunt's diagnosis wasn't the first time cancer had struck her family. Her grandmother on her mother's side died of cancer when her mother was five years old, an event that affected her mother for the rest of her life. Her mother, Anna Mae, was raised by her two sisters. The oldest sister, Sylvia, was diagnosed with cancer in her forties and died within five years. What young Julie did not know at the time of Sylvia's death was that each of the three sisters, one after the next, would be diagnosed with breast cancer in their early forties and die approximately five years after the diagnosis.

When Flossie was diagnosed, Anna Mae became visibly depressed. It was torturous for her to have to watch her second and last sister suffer and die of cancer, and she began to fear that her turn was coming soon. Julie, who still strongly identified with her mother, felt her sadness and fears right along with her. Her aunt Flossie had a mastectomy and began a chemotherapy regimen that would prove too weak a treatment to fight the aggressive cancer that with unrelenting ferocity has ravaged this family.

At the same time of her aunt's mastectomy, Julie noticed her own body beginning to develop.

> *That's the age when you're trying to be popular in school, when you're worried about being pretty, and when body image becomes important. I had very conflicting issues about my breasts. On the one hand, I was happy they were growing, and on the other hand, I thought, these are going to bring me problems, and problems I won't be able to control. My breasts are growing and at the same time I'm worried about losing them. I had no control over how big they were going to grow and what they were going to do on their own. I always thought that if I kept them smaller, it would be easier to detect a cancer and I would have a better chance of surviving or there wouldn't be enough tissue for it to form.*

So she took control in the only way she knew. "I remember when I was in ninth grade, a girlfriend told me she wanted to be thin, and to accomplish that, she threw up. So I said, 'How do you do that?' and she showed me by sticking two fingers down her throat. That's when my eating disorder started. The ironic thing is that my friend stopped doing it, but it stayed with me for sixteen years." From the age of thirteen to twenty-nine, Julie alternated between starving herself, the eating disorder known as anorexia, and bingeing and purging, called bulimia.

Eating disorders are not typically caused by one event or influence but by a number of factors, such as personality traits and self-esteem, the family environment, parental styles, and external events. But experts have recognized some similarities in the women who tend to have eating disorders. Typically, young women who develop anorexia have overprotective, over-involved mothers, explains body-image specialist Adrienne Ressler, from

The Renfrew Center, an eating disorder clinic in Coconut Creek, Florida. In response, daughters are overly dependent and obedient young women who have difficulty asserting themselves in healthy ways.

Julie seemed to fit this description. She had been born prematurely and contracted meningitis, a bacterial infection of the spinal cord, which left her with a hearing disability. Children with disabilities tend to be more dependent on their mothers for their connection to the outside world, particularly in their younger years (the phenomenon was even more pronounced when Julie was growing up in the 1970s). "When we went to family gatherings or any group things, it was hard for me to understand things. So I always sat by my mom's side, and I never had to worry about missing anything because she always repeated things for me," explains Julie, who says she can hear some sounds but not distinguish words. Until seventh grade, Julie also depended on her mother, a schoolteacher, for social companionship, because her speech was not clear when she was young. "After school, I just came home and spent a lot of time with my mother. No one except my mother had the stamina to try to understand me," says Julie, who today, after fifteen years of speech therapy, speaks with mild imperfections.

Eating disorders are also about regaining control. "When a young girl feels that her life is out of control, she may take on an eating disorder as a way of controlling things," says Ressler. "Certainly, fear of illness or fear of a parent dying is a very out-of-control feeling." Typically, in women with eating disorders, there's also a lack of openness in the family to real conflicts, so children cope with their feelings on their own. Though Julie could confide in her mother about anything, and the two had a seemingly open relationship, when it came to cancer, her mother became stoic. When Flossie was diagnosed with cancer, Julie's mother shut down emotionally. "I couldn't talk to my mother about my aunt dying because I picked up on her fear and I knew it was too painful for her to talk about," says Julie. But Julie was panicking herself. She was losing her aunt, who was like a second mother to her, and in the back of her mind, she feared that the same fate would befall her own mother. Adding to all the illness-related problems, Julie's parents had recently divorced. "I couldn't tell my family I was hurting, so I kept it in. But now, after years of therapy, I understand that the throwing up was a way of trying to get rid of the hurt feelings. It became my coping mechanism. It was the only thing I could control. It was the way I could survive at that time," says Julie.

> *I began by bingeing when I got home from school. I had an hour or so before my mom got home from work, so I binged on anything that was in the house. I binged on things I didn't like. It didn't matter what I ate; the point was to stuff myself so I could throw up. I ate with my hands, taking everything and stuffing it in. I had this feeling of numbing out, like I was in a trance state. It wasn't about tasting the food or enjoying it; it was how much can I consume that I can get out. It was all about getting it out.*

Though eating disorders begin with the feeling of power and control for girls, they quickly become a compulsion, such as drug use, and the girls lose control. "When you have an eating disorder, you appear strong on the outside, but you're falling apart on the inside," says Julie. None of her friends knew she was doing her after-school binge-and-purge routine. She was an otherwise social person, with high grades and good behavior. It was a quiet rebellion, acting *in* rather than acting *out.*

Maybe the rebellion would have passed if her life stabilized, but things only got worse. By the time she was sixteen years old, her aunt Flossie's cancer had metastasized to her brain. The tumors began to affect her aunt's memory, her mind, and her behavior, to the point that she no longer seemed like the same person. Eventually her aunt suffered complete dementia. "She was more like a vegetable," recalls Julie. That year, 1979, Julie's mother, at the age of forty-two, was diagnosed with breast cancer.

"I remember going to visit my mother in the hospital, where she was having a biopsy of a suspicious lump. She was lying in bed, and she told me it was malignant, and I cried hysterically. I was so afraid of the final outcome, which was that I would lose her like I was losing my aunt," says Julie. Her mother had a mastectomy, followed by chemotherapy, but it was hard for anyone in the family to hold out hope after witnessing two sisters lose the battle with cancer. Two years later, Flossie died, taking with her Anna Mae's own will to live.

"I said to my mom, you have us to live for," says Julie, referring to herself and her older sister and brother. "She said, 'You don't understand; I've lost my family. It's not enough.'" Seeing her mother give up on life was more than Julie could handle. The eating disorder escalated. "I would binge and purge eight times a day. I'd go out to buy junk food, come home, and eat my whole stash. Just as other people would go buy drugs, I'd go buy ice cream and cookies." When she cycled back to anorexia, she wouldn't eat for weeks, priding herself on getting by on a carrot stick or piece of celery. "When I became anorexic, I lost a lot of weight, and my breasts would get smaller. I even lost my period once for several months. I'm five feet five and normally I'd weigh 125 pounds, but I went down to 100 pounds when I was anorexic. When I was bulimic, I'd go back up to 155 pounds. I have clothes in my closet that range in size from 4 to 12." Julie believes her mother knew about her eating disorder but didn't know how to confront her. When Julie would try to hint at her eating problem, her mother wouldn't grasp the severity of it. "She would say, 'I know you're a vegetarian. We'll get you more vegetables,'" recalls Julie. She couldn't face it. "She had her own issues she was dealing with," says Julie.

"My mom would come home from chemotherapy and be nauseated; she wouldn't talk about it. She was like a martyr. 'I'm not going to share this with anybody. I'm not going to let anyone know I'm in pain.' She would never allow us to be the caregivers. I wanted to take the pain away and I couldn't, so I went and binged and threw up. I felt so helpless." Watching a mother suffer the fatigue and nausea of chemotherapy, the embarrassment of mastectomy or baldness, and other painful symptoms is almost worse than dealing with these symptoms yourself. "When it's your own illness, you often can generate ways to get some sense of control over these things," says University of Vermont's Bruce Compas. "When you're watching somebody else suffer, you don't have that sense that you can do something to change it and make it better, so it's a helpless situation." Julie's mother eventually had reconstructive surgery but was unhappy with the way it looked.

> *The surgery wasn't good at the time. I thought it looked awful. She used to take baths, and I would see her chest all the time. She would never say anything, and I remember feeling horrified of what she had to go through. I felt almost a survivor's guilt. I have my breasts and she doesn't. Well, an eating disorder is the perfect way of dealing with that. Deep down I was thinking, even though I don't have breast cancer, I'm still going to suffer with my mother.*

Her mother's cancer was eradicated, and life returned to normal for several years. Julie went off to college in New York City. "I wanted to get away, and pretend that nothing was wrong with my mother, that she would be fine and I would be fine," says Julie. But the eating disorder persisted. "In college, my roommate didn't know I had the eating disorder. She had junk food all over the place. I was very thin when I started college, the thinnest I'd ever been. But I started bingeing on my roommate's food. I would wait till she was in class to binge. Or I'd go into other people's food at night, and then I'd go out shopping in the middle of the night to replace it before they woke up," says Julie.

During her sophomore year, Julie swung back into a starvation phase, which was when she fainted in front of her dorm room. Fearing she would end up in the hospital if she didn't seek help, Julie called a counselor on campus and put herself into therapy. "Then I called my mother and told her I was seeing a therapist because I hadn't eaten in a week, and if I didn't eat, I was going to die," says Julie. Her mother drove up to New York City and attended a therapy session with Julie, where they talked about feelings that had been suppressed for so long. "What really made a difference for me was that for the first time, I felt like my mom was scrutinizing herself. She said, 'Is this my fault?' It's not that I thought it was her fault, but for her to be open to the possibility that there was something she could have done differently to help me cope meant the world to me. She knew that I was telling her something she needed to hear, and she was listening. It was one of my most memorable times with her. I was so vulnerable about my illness, and she gave complete compassion and support, and wanted to know what she could do to make me better," say Julie.

"That was the beginning of my journey to being healed. When she came and did that, I knew it might be a tremendous struggle, but one day I might not have this eating disorder," says Julie. It did, in fact, take another ten years for her to fully recover. "Like being an alcoholic, you're never over it. I'd get a feeling that I'd want to binge and say, 'I'm not going to do it today,' and I'd be fine for a day, then something would trigger an emotion and I'd do it again." It was particularly difficult to cure herself while living through the advanced stages of her mother's cancer.

On Julie's twentieth birthday, during a visit home from college, Julie was informed by her sister Lori that her mother's cancer had metastasized. "My mom came downstairs and saw me crying and said, 'What's wrong?' I said, 'I know you're dying.' I think she was stunned. It hadn't registered with her. She said, 'Just calm down.' It really was never discussed after that. I had to go through the whole process on my own."

Her mother's physical and mental health took a dramatic turn for the worse. The cancer spread to her brain, and began to affect her mother's mind, as it had her aunt Flossie's. She began forgetting things and acting erratically, and then, like an Alzheimer's patient, it was as if she was not there at all. She remained like that for almost two years.

> When it metastasized to her brain, I was throwing up constantly. I was in so much pain. It was like being in limbo; my mom's no longer here, but her body's here. I wanted her to die at that point, she was in so much pain and she didn't have any quality of life. She was living in the hospital. I remember one Christmas Eve I went to visit her. The nurses had put her in a chair in the hallway by the nurses' station for some reason. She was sitting there alone. She had her wig on backwards. She had Jell-O dripping from her face and had a bib on like she was two years old. I wanted to scream, 'This is somebody's mother! This

> *is somebody's teacher! What are you doing, walking by her*
> *and not even cleaning her mouth? How inhumane can you*
> *be?' But I was young, so I didn't say anything. I went*
> *home and threw up instead.*

Her mother died three months before Julie was to graduate from college. Julie managed to finish what she needed to do to get her bachelor's degree, though her grades dropped and she didn't attend graduation. Soon after her mother died, she decided to move to Southern California. "It was much easier for me to start over somewhere else than to be there with all the memories and reminders of her," says Julie. Though the move helped in the grieving process, it did not help alleviate her fears of getting cancer herself.

Julie and Lori and their first cousin Staci, Flossie's daughter, were all keenly aware of their family tree. It's as saturated with breast cancer as can be. "When we were in our twenties, we used to joke that since cancer hits the women in our family in their forties, we had twenty years that we didn't have to worry about it," says Julie. But they were worried. When Julie was twenty-four, she found a lump the size of a golf ball in her breast. "I was panicked, so I called my sister at four in the morning, hysterical. She had to coach me through this," she recalls. "I remember being angry at my mom for not teaching me how to handle it. She never talked about what it felt like going through everything. She didn't want to hurt us, but she didn't help us either," says Julie. The lump was a benign cyst, but Julie had it removed anyway. "I told the doctor, I cannot live with this in my body," says Julie.

The three women lived with a fear of cancer for many years until they heard about the new test for a mutation in the BRCA gene that's linked to breast cancer and ovarian cancer. Lori and Staci both decided to get tested. They both were married and had two children and decided that if they tested positive for the BRCA gene mutation, they would each have two preventive surgeries, a prophylactic mastectomy with reconstruction and a prophylactic oophorectomy (removal of the ovaries). It was the only way they felt they would live to be older than the last generation of women—past the age of fifty. Julie, being single, felt she was not ready to lose her breasts and her reproductive organs, so she opted out of the test. Lori and Staci did test positive for the mutation, and both went through with the surgeries. Julie still had a 50-50 chance that she hadn't inherited the gene. But the fear continued to plague her, and by the time she turned thirty-four, though she was still single, she decided that knowing if she carried the mutation was better than living with the uncertainty, even if she wasn't going to have preventive surgery. "I knew that the fear was going to run me anyway, so I might as well face it," says Julie.

She had her blood drawn, and about four weeks later (the test is labor intensive), she returned to receive her results. She had asked a breast cancer survivor to go with her so that she'd have a positive role model for support if she learned she had the mutation. Julie tested positive, and despite her family history, she was stunned. The risk counselor estimated that her risk of getting breast cancer was between 65 and 85 percent. "I freaked out when I first found out. I thought, this is going to change my life. How am I going to handle this?" says Julie. Once she got over the shock of the news, however, it became a catalyst in her life. It was as if she had a near death experience, which is not entirely inaccurate. "It has been the best thing I ever found out," says Julie. "Now I live my life completely the way I want to. I used to want to please my sister, so I'd do whatever she thought was right. She was always more pragmatic than me. I was finally able to stand up to her for the first time in my life." Julie bought a new car and got a more fulfilling job as a school counselor for special education children. She had become a therapist because she felt she owed her life to the therapist who helped her recover from the eating disorder, and she wanted to give back to others; she works with children because that is what her mother did. "My goal is to write children's books," says Julie, who now lives her life with a sense of purpose. "I also want to start a support group for women who have the breast cancer gene mutation, because there is no place for us to go, and my big dream is to open a healing center for sick mothers."

She still worries about cancer but believes that she won't die from it. She has done everything she possibly can to prevent this outcome. She has stuck to her decision against prophylactic mastectomy. Instead, she gets a mammogram twice a year, sees a breast specialist every four months, gets blood tests regularly, maintains a totally organic diet, rarely drinks alcohol, and takes yoga. "I always knew that this was how I wanted to handle it, but the test made it an absolute commitment to do so. Suddenly, it became a matter of my surviving," says Julie. Most important, getting tested cured her once and for all of her eating disorder, largely because she had begun to take control of her health and her emotions in more healthy ways. "When I was really into my eating disorder, I couldn't remember a time when I didn't binge and throw up," says Julie. "Now I can't remember the last time I did it. I never thought it would flip that way."

6

ANGER AND LOVE

"All of a sudden, both of our walls came down and we were able to talk at a nice equal level and not fight, not get defensive, and not get angry."

Stephanie Oster, 35

STEPHANIE OSTER
NEW YORK, NEW YORK

*W*hen Stephanie Oster turned nineteen, she packed up her things and left home. She didn't leave to go to college; she didn't leave to take a decent job to sustain her; she left to get away. She left angry, fed up with her family, and thought that this was the end of her relationship with her mother.

At the age of thirty, Stephanie came home again, to Long Island, New York, where she had grown up, summoned by her mother who was dying of breast cancer.

Sitting under a tree in New York City's Central Park, a few blocks from her apartment, Stephanie, with blue-green eyes and straight brown hair streaked with blond, speaks in a low, soft voice about what made her leave home. "When I was very young, my mother and I had a special connection and we both knew that. We were very close and had an intuitive sense about each other," says Stephanie. But after her parents got a divorce, when Stephanie was twelve, the circumstances of their lives chipped away at their connection. Her mother, who had been miserable in marriage, began enjoying life for the first time, going out on dates and socializing. But in so doing, she often left Stephanie and her two sisters to fend for themselves, sometimes for entire weekends. "My mother was pretty negligent at that time," recalls Stephanie. Her mother, Jeannine, was not there to perform her maternal role, such as asking Stephanie whether she'd finished her homework, inquiring about her extracurricular activities, or encouraging her to apply to college. She was also not there for the necessities—to cook dinner and go grocery shopping. "I remember several times when I had to go over to my father's house, who lived nearby, and borrow the car to go buy toilet paper and milk because my mom didn't do any shopping that week," says Stephanie. After her older sister left for college, Stephanie became saddled with the job of taking care of her little sister, who was six years younger. Stephanie cooked, she cleaned, and she tried to provide her younger sister with the kind of guidance that she was deprived of herself, but it was too much for a teenager to handle. "When my sister was old enough, I finally took off. I thought, I don't need to be raising a family at this age," she recalls. "I was really resentful of all that I missed out on. I didn't think my parents were good parents and I remember saying to myself, I don't need them, I'm not coming home again."

Stephanie moved to Massachusetts and enrolled in a community college, but she eventually left for California, forgoing college. Instead she worked and traveled a lot of traveling throughout the world, speaking only occasionally by phone to her mother. It was during one of these conversations that her mother told her she had found a lump and it was malignant. "I remember I was slightly alarmed, but my mother always had this way of leading us to believe that we never had to worry. I said, 'Do you want me to come home?' She said, 'I'm fine. It's nothing,' in this special phone voice she had that was very upbeat." Stephanie's mother had a lumpectomy but did not have chemotherapy or radiation. She was wary of these treatments, partly because she had a friend who had died of complications from chemotherapy and also because she was a strong believer in alternative medicine. Within a couple of years, her mother found another lump, had a second lumpectomy, then discovered a third lump, at which point she underwent a mastectomy. Stephanie, still estranged, never came home for any of these surgeries.

By this time, Stephanie had married and moved back East, to Nantucket, an island off the coast of Massachusetts, where she and her husband took seasonal jobs—she as a hair colorist, he as a carpenter—so they could save enough money to travel the rest of the year. But one day, Stephanie got a call from one of her mother's friends, who said, "Your mother's really sick. You ought to come home."

"I guess it was the wake-up call I needed," says Stephanie, who packed up and went home, thinking that she'd stay for the weekend. "I came home and my mother was thin and frail. I just had no idea. Because of her happy phone voice, I didn't know how sick she was." Neither of her sisters were aware of their mother's condition either. Stephanie stayed for a month to take care of her mother, and the two women, brought together for the first time since Stephanie was a teenager, began to mend the relationship that had been broken so many years ago.

It was, however, a slow, contentious process between mother and daughter, a pulling in and pushing away. It began simply by their being forced together, required to communicate with each other to make it through the day. "I didn't know what to do first, so I began helping around the house and doing the shopping, because she was too tired to do these things," says Stephanie. Her younger sister was in college in California, and her older sister, though living in New York City, let Stephanie bear the brunt of the work.

In the beginning, I did what I had to do, all the practical things, but I acted kind of cold. I was really short-tempered with her. We fell back into old patterns of having these shouting matches. I got frustrated with her because she was never a good listener, she has always drifted in and out of our conversations. That pushed some old buttons. Because she didn't listen well, I never felt like she really knew me. When I moved home, she thought she knew who

I was, and she'd make these big generalizations about me, and I wanted to say to her, "You don't know me at all. I have not been present for the last ten years."

I had to maintain a certain distance. She wanted so badly to be my mother, to have that mother-daughter let's cuddle up, let's be best friends and go out to lunch relationship. I just resisted her for so long. I could be there for her, because, yes, she was the woman who gave birth to me and took care of me as a child, and yes, I could relate to her as a friend, but I couldn't be cuddly. That just hadn't been our relationship for so long. But there was definitely a mutual caring, just my being there, she knew I was there for a reason. I couldn't say, "I'm here because I love you and I'm here because I care about you." But the fact was, I was there and she knew that.

Stephanie and Jeannine fell into a routine, eating meals together, watching television during the day or videos in the evenings, and as time passed, they started to open up with each other. "We began to have really great conversations. All of a sudden the wall came down and we were able to talk at a nice equal level and not fight, not get defensive, and not get angry," says Stephanie. "I told her how angry I was with her, and she apologized. And I tried to understand things from her perspective." Her mother explained what was going on with her after the divorce, how she was trying to meet new people and create a life for herself. Stephanie tried hard to listen objectively, to view her mother as just another woman, like a friend confiding in another friend. "Even though the little girl in me was still angry, the adult in me began to understand. I thought, yeah, I know what it's like to be single. It's hard out there."

Stephanie's mother also told her more about herself before she got married, what her own parents were like, and she talked about Stephanie's father. "For the first time, she spoke about him realistically, like there were fond moments and there were bad moments. It wasn't that post-divorce, 'your father's a shit' thing. I felt like I got to know her through her stories of her relationships with my father, her parents, and other people."

Cancer or any serious illness can allow mothers and daughters to transcend their issues. "Especially when cancer is terminal, both the mother and the daughter have the chance to say to each other things that have never been said before," says psychologist Evelyn Bassoff. "There is an enormous amount of suffering with cancer, but there is also the chance for amazing growth. Everything is put in perspective, the problems that cause rifts between mothers and daughters can be let go, and something very meaningful can happen."

Stephanie and her mother began to feel their relationship developing into something much more than either of them had imagined. "We both really tried to make up for the lost time. I told her more about myself and my relationship with my husband, and the problems we were having. When she got sick, she became more insightful, because she took the time to think about things, instead of answering with a cliché," says Stephanie. Jeannine listened and for the first time she began to see who her daughter was. "Every daughter wants to be known and loved for who she is by her mother," says Bassoff. "The greatest gift a mother can give a daughter is the gift of approval, that feeling of motherly approval that empowers the daughter for her whole life."

Jeannine decided to go to an alternative treatment center in Mexico that treated cancer patients with strict organic diets and nutritional supplements. She stayed for a month. Stephanie felt frustrated that her mother wouldn't try chemotherapy. "I tried to have an influence on her, but my mother was very educated about this. She had read every book on cancer that you can imagine. So I also wanted to support her in whatever she wanted to do because I knew that if she didn't believe in what she was doing, it wouldn't work," says Stephanie. Her mother's latest choice, however, may not have been a good one. "When I picked her up at the airport, she just looked like a bag of bones. I got really scared. For the first time I thought, wow, my mom's really sick." At that moment, Stephanie decided to move back home. There was no question in her mind that she should come home and take care of her mother full-time. Her husband stayed in Nantucket and came to visit her on weekends, an arrangement that put a strain on their already troubled relationship. When their mothers are very sick from cancer, many daughters see it as an opportunity to leave a less than wonderful relationship or even a job. When suddenly forced to decide between spending their time with a dying mother or spending time with someone who has not made them very happy, the choice is clear.

Stephanie's days were devoted to preparing her mother's remedies, such as organic juices and soaps, trying to get her to eat, and cleaning up. She'd leave just enough time to go for a quick run and then to the gym, a physical release that helped maintain her sanity. In the summer, she'd go to the beach at four in the afternoon, dive into a bracing wave, then swim along the shoreline for about an hour. Stephanie's mother had a close male friend who would stop by every day and bring flowers, food, and videos, or he'd take her to the beach. "My mother never fell romantically in love with him, but in the end, she really loved him and knew she was lucky to have him." For Stephanie, his presence was a relief, as he was the only person who helped ease the caregiving burden. Otherwise, Stephanie was alone. Her two sisters were not particularly helpful.

> *My older sister, though she lived close by, was kind of in denial. She avoided coming over, and when she did, she stayed for maybe an hour, then split. My younger sister helped out a lot, but she was in college in California. She had come home for about a month during the summer, but in September, when school started up again, my mother told her she should go back to school, so she did. I was surprised that she didn't take a leave from school. I guess my sisters did what they could. Not everyone drops everything, and I can't expect them to. I wasn't trying to be a martyr either, but I couldn't see not doing it. I think I was the only one in the family that really knew my mother was dying.*

The role of caregiver has traditionally fallen on the daughter, but that can be a problem for daughters who don't want to take on that role. "For some, taking care of the mother's body feels too uncomfortable," says Bassoff. "But those daughters who don't come to their mother's aid may feel guilty because of the traditional pressures. They shouldn't feel guilty, as long as the mother is cared for either by other family members or by a professional nurse."

Guilt is hard to avoid when a parent is dying, and Stephanie wasn't spared the gnawing emotion. "I have guilt because I was selfish at times with her. Even though I was there for her, sometimes I wasn't really there. I got resentful because I had to give up my life, so I wasn't always the warmest person," recalls Stephanie, a memory that's so painful to her that her eyes start to tear. Taking care of a sick mother, which comes with the emotional trauma of a role reversal, the unrequited giving of oneself, the physical exhaustion, and the fear of mother dying, is one of the most stressful and demanding experiences in life. Needless to say, many daughters are not always as wonderful at it as they'd like to be. "The wish is to be an all-loving, all-patient caregiver when the reality is much more like you're angry, you're frustrated, you become impatient, and you dislike aspects of your mother's personality," says Allison Ross, a psychologist in private practice in New York City. "These negative feelings, though normal, can leave the daughters feeling very guilty."

> *There were definitely times when I lost patience. I'd yell at her and get mean. I was angry at her at times for being sick. So we had these shouting fights, and then I looked at her and thought, oh my God, she's so frail. She can't fight with me. I would forget she's not like the mother I used to fight with. We used to really go at it. Then when she was sick, she pushed those old buttons and I fell back into those old patterns and looked at her, and she was so defeated. I felt terrible. There are things that I did that I wish I hadn't. I did the best I could, which was not perfect.*

For about six months, Jeannine's health was slowly deteriorating, but to Stephanie, her mother seemed to be in denial. "We never had that 'When I die' conversation. There was only one time when she said, 'I'm scared I might be dying.' She was so terrified, she was shaking. I held her in my arms like a little baby. A daughter can't say to her mother, 'Yeah, Mom, you *are* dying.' I just said, 'I'm here, don't worry. I won't leave you.'" By this time, there was no trace of the anger that had come between mother and daughter in the past.

One afternoon, when Stephanie and her mother were watching TV, they saw an ad for the Cancer Treatment Centers of America, a center in Illinois that combines chemotherapy treatments with alternative therapies such as individualized diets, nutritional supplements, treatments believed to stimulate the immune system, physical therapy, massage, and psychological and spiritual support. Her mother, beginning to feel keenly aware that her health was quickly deteriorating, decided that this holistic approach to chemotherapy might be a good compromise. Stephanie called the toll-free number and booked a flight for the two of them that afternoon. The call added a year to her life, a very good year. The physician immediately put her mother on feeding tubes because she was suffering from malnutrition. At this center, oncologists typically dole out chemotherapy incrementally over a period of five days, rather than dousing the body with the noxious chemicals all at once. Because of the gentler dose, Jeannine never lost her hair or suffered any nausea. For several months, her mother would fly out to the center and stay for a week of treatment. Stephanie always felt a bit of relief when she left, a sense of freedom that for seven days she could live her life and not worry about her mother's care.

While taking care of her mother, Stephanie came to the decision that she wouldn't return to her husband. "The cancer definitely brought my marriage to a finish, although it would have gotten there anyway. We had married very quickly after we met, in three months, and I think that after a few years he had fallen out of love with me, but I had been fighting it. Now I was dealing with my mother dying. It was the most significant thing that had ever happened to me. I realized that saving my marriage just wasn't the most important thing in my life." It's not uncommon for a mother's life-threatening illness to prompt a daughter to take inventory of her own life and to deal with issues she had been avoiding. As Stephanie's mother started getting better with her monthly excursions to Illinois, Stephanie rented an apartment in New York City and began a new life.

Her mother's chemotherapy stalled the progression of the cancer for about a year, and it was the best year that she and Stephanie had together. Jeannine felt well enough to go out and live her life again, spending weekends in the city with Stephanie, or her boyfriend would take her to shows and dinner. Stephanie and her younger sister conspired to take their mother to France, where she was born and had lived as a little girl. Her mother hadn't been back to Europe since her family emigrated to the United States. "We celebrated her birthday at a fabulous restaurant in Paris. My mother had been on all these special diets for so long, but that night she ate and drank whatever she wanted and had a wonderful time at it. The next day, we drove out to the country, to Lorraine, and went to the apartment where she was born. It was on a little main street above a store. We went to the town hall and got her birth certificate. Her clearest memory was of a house in the country, where a woman would take care of her. We were driving around looking for it when my mother yelled, 'Stop the car! I know this place!' It was a forest where she and her father used to take walks, and she remembered the smell of pine. We walked in the forest, and she closed her eyes, and it brought back all these memories."

The trip was just in time. About three or four months after she had stopped going for chemotherapy, her mother began to have trouble with her back. Tests revealed that the cancer had metastasized to her spine. She went back to the hospital in Illinois for more chemotherapy treatments. They sent her home with a morphine patch for the pain, but after a few days, she became confused and disoriented, so she flew back to the hospital. Within a couple of days, the doctor called Stephanie, who was back in New York, and told her that her mother had pneumonia. "I hung up the phone and it took me about five minutes to realize that she's not going to make it. I said, all right, I gotta go. Mom's going to die; I gotta go. I called my sisters and said we have to go out there. I was hysterical and in control at the same time. By the time we got there, my mother was very confused and was already on oxygen." Jeannine didn't recognize Stephanie's older sisters. They realized that they were too late, that their mother had already begun to die.

"When the doctors were taking her into the operating room to put her on a ventilator to help her breathe, and I knew she wouldn't be able to speak to us ever again, I leaned over to her, I whispered in her ear, 'I love you, Mom.' She said 'I love you too, Stephanie.' Those were the last words we spoke. I was so surprised because I was positive that she had no idea what was going on around her, but even in her confusion, when I spoke to her, she knew exactly who I was. I think she really knew only me; she didn't know what to do with my other sisters. Despite all the distance between us and the years we were apart, I was able to create a meaningful relationship with my mother. I'm almost positive it had to do with her being ill. I don't think we would ever have had that relationship if she weren't sick. It was something I never expected to have with her. It was that mother-daughter thing that she wanted, and much more."

7

DEPRESSION AND FEAR

"I'm convinced that I'm going to get breast cancer in my mid-forties just like my mother, just like her mother."
Jennifer Harrington, 29

JENNIFER HARRINGTON
BALTIMORE, MARYLAND

"*I* had gotten to a point where I couldn't really function," says Jennifer Harrington, twenty-nine, her voice soft, like a hurt child's. "I was bursting into tears at random. I felt overwhelmed by everything. I'm a graduate student and I'm supposed to be writing my dissertation, and I just had a really hard time making any progress on it." Jennifer would sit in her study, a small bedroom lined with bookshelves from floor to ceiling, and try to concentrate on her writing, but all she could think about was that her mother was dying. "I spent my days either lying in bed worrying or staring at my computer screen, trying to write, but worrying," she says. "Even taking the dog for a walk or doing the dishes or making dinner was difficult for me to do."

Jennifer is five feet one, her body more sturdy than petite, her face broad and friendly. She is a political scientist living in Baltimore, and was twenty-six and only a few months from her wedding day when her mother was diagnosed with breast cancer. The news, in fact, came on the day of Jennifer's bridal shower.

That morning, she couldn't understand why her mother, Mickey, seemed so frantic while cleaning the house. She had been vacuuming and mopping with such an intensity that she seemed like a Judy Davis character on speed. "I thought she was nervous because it was supposed to be a surprise shower even though I knew about it," says Jennifer. But then she overheard her mother talking on the phone to Jennifer's aunt, saying that she had a lump biopsied and it looked pretty bad. "I guess you can say, I went deeply into denial. I didn't even process what I heard," says Jennifer.

The next day, Mickey, who was forty-six, called Jennifer to confirm that it was malignant. "It was my worst nightmare come true. Breast cancer is something I've been aware of for as long as I can remember," says Jennifer. She knew as a young girl that her grandmother died of the disease when her mother was only eleven years old. "I can't remember a time when I wasn't aware that my mother had a really high risk. I can't remember a time when I didn't expect her to get cancer," she says.

It was a particularly scary prospect for Jennifer, given her family situation. She is an only child, her parents had divorced when she was twelve years old, and she and her mother had grown extremely close because it was just the two of them. Today, they live in different states, Jennifer in Maryland, her mother four hours away in Pennsylvania, but they call each other on the phone at least once a day and talk about everything from literature and politics to the minutiae of their lives. Recently, as Jennifer has begun to establish her own household, they have more in common and speak more as friends than as mother and daughter. "It's not that I'm that dependent on her; I just really like her, and I like being able to call her whenever I want and being able to ask her for advice about things," says Jennifer. "We both really enjoy reading, and we both love pets. I've just started gardening, and she's an avid gardener. I like to call her and say 'The bottom leaves on my tomatoes are turning yellow. What should I do?'"

Mickey had been reluctant to tell her daughter about the cancer because Jennifer was scheduled to fly to San Francisco to deliver a major paper at a national conference of political scientists at the same time that her mother had scheduled the lumpectomy. "This paper was based on four months of field work I did in Cairo, it was the subject of my dissertation, and all of a sudden it seemed so incredibly irrelevant. I wanted to cancel my trip and just be with my mother," says Jennifer. Her mother, as any mother would do, insisted that Jennifer not miss this career opportunity, so Jennifer kept her plans and flew to San Francisco. But through her whole trip, except during her actual speech, fears about her mother—in the hospital, in surgery, in recovery—intruded, interrupted, and fully occupied her mind.

If breast cancer hits a family when a daughter is striking out on her own, trying to launch her career and create her own family and her own home, these adventures can be tainted by feelings of indifference, insecurity, and sadness, says psychologist Evelyn Bassoff. This is a time when having a secure home to fall back on can give us the courage to push ahead. It's a time when the mother is supposed to be the guide, the unconditional supporter, the person with whom we compare and contrast ourselves as we make our way through the world. But when a mother is sick, there is less joy in these endeavors, as the prospect of reaching life's milestones without her begins to feel as real as a lump beneath your fingertips.

The milestone Jennifer was approaching was her wedding, but with her mother's breast cancer looming, it was causing her anxiety—more so than the run-of-the-mill stress that leads up to the big event. "I was really upset about the cancer, but it seemed as if it had been caught early. It was under three centimeters, and it wasn't in her lymph nodes," says Jennifer. That meant her mother had a five-year survival rate of about 84 percent. "Still, I tend to think the worst, so I vacillated between feeling like the world was ending and thinking it was going to be okay. In the process, the wedding itself just seemed so totally unimportant," she adds. It turned out that the tissue surrounding the lump that was removed wasn't completely free of malignant cells—in medical speak, the margins weren't clear—so the doctors recommended that Mickey undergo a mastectomy, right after the wedding.

Jennifer and her husband, Brian, departed on their honeymoon reluctantly, again at the insistence of her mother. This would be the second surgery that Jennifer would miss. She was counting. From the quaint bed and breakfast in Maine, where they were supposed to be basking in their new marital status, Jennifer made sure to call her mother to see how the surgery and her recuperation were going. Brian, whose own father had been battling cancer for many years, understood Jennifer's need to call home. He was used to illness interrupting the normal flow of life.

Upon their return from Maine, the newlyweds endured a series of blows that would nudge Jennifer over the emotional edge. A couple of days after they returned from Maine, when tooling around Baltimore, they were in a car accident, which totaled their car and left Jennifer with a sprained neck and a face cut and bruised from the air bag. "I'm five foot one and am one of those people who can get killed by an air bag," she says. She couldn't visit her mother until she was able to extract a rental car from her insurance company. When she finally arrived in Pennsylvania about a week later, Jennifer accompanied her mother to the doctor to discuss the treatment and the results of a CAT scan. Her mother had asked the oncologist to do the scan of her liver, because her own mother's cancer had spread to the liver. Her doctor thought it was totally unnecessary because the cancer wasn't that advanced, but he accommodated her request.

"When he came in to talk to us about the results, he looked stunned. He was pale. He said the cancer was in her liver, and he didn't know why and it shouldn't have been, but it was," says Jennifer. "It was such a blow. All of a sudden, within a blink of an eye, my mother went from being lucky that she caught it early to having metastatic cancer. My mother was shocked because the cancer should not have spread at all and certainly not to her liver. But she's a fighter and wanted to know exactly what the battle plan was and wanted to take the most aggressive course of treatment possible." Even though Jennifer always lived with the fear that her mother would get breast cancer, she never assumed it was going to be as aggressive as it was. To keep herself sane, she had always held out hope that medical science would keep her mother alive, but now this news wiped any hope away.

The oncologist doubled her mother's chemo treatment from three months to six. "Watching my mother endure the effects of

chemotherapy during those months was torture and only solidi-
fied my concerns about her," says Jennifer. One incident in particular had a lasting effect on her. Jennifer, Brian, and her mother
decided to drive to Atlanta for a Thanksgiving family reunion at
her mother's sister's house. It was right after her mother's second
chemotherapy treatment. Her mother hadn't had a bad reaction
to the first round of chemo, but this time, she got very ill—about
halfway to Atlanta. She had intense fatigue, debilitating diarrhea,
and vomiting. When they arrived in Atlanta, she had to go to the
emergency room twice because of dehydration. "This was the
first time I had ever seen my mother really sick and weak, and it
made her vulnerability to this disease all the more real and vivid
in my mind, and it profoundly disturbed and scared me," recalls
Jennifer.

Despite that one setback, her mother pushed ahead with
optimism, but Jennifer was encumbered by pessimism and a
sense of hopelessness. She could barely deal with the rapid accel-
eration and the worsened prognosis of her mother's disease. "All
I could think of was my father-in-law's prophetic words about his
own lung cancer: 'As long as it doesn't spread to the liver. A
metastasis to the liver is a death sentence.'" Of course, that's
exactly where her mother's cancer had spread. "Seeing my father-
in-law and my mother in such bad shape and knowing that what
was killing him—the metastasis to the liver—was what my mother had was overwhelming," she says.

Jennifer fell into a depression, first not doing any work,
then not being able to do simple day-to-day tasks. She would sit
at her desk, gazing at the bulletin board over her desk that was
plastered with cards and pictures. Her eyes often set on one picture, the snapshot of Mickey helping Jennifer with her veil on the
day of her wedding.

> *What I mostly "looked" at was a picture in my head
> that I saw in a magazine years ago. It was a picture of a
> woman who was dying of breast cancer. She looked like a
> concentration camp victim—virtually skin and bones. Her
> daughter was helping her get up out of bed. I often think
> about that picture—without meaning to—and realize that*

this is very likely my mother's fate. No one should have to die that way.

Her depression evolved into fear. She was afraid that her mother was going to die and suddenly feared for her own life.

Even though my grandmother died of cancer, I didn't start worrying about myself until my mother was diagnosed. I felt that generation struck out, now it's this generation's turn. I became convinced that my breasts were going to kill me. For a while, I was obsessively checking for lumps and hoping that I'd find one so I could just get it over with. I knew that some day there'd be one there, so I'd rather it was today than some unspecified time in the future. I'm convinced that I'm going to get breast cancer in my mid-forties just like my mother, just like her mother.

Whatever the cause of a mother's death, most of us think that we will die at the same age that our mother's do, whether she dies when she is seventy-five or forty-five. It's an irrational belief, but it's very powerful. When a mother gets cancer or dies at an early age, that idea weighs even more heavily on us, says Bassoff, adding, "As a daughter approaches that age, she becomes very nervous about her mortality."

February 7, 1997, was a bad day in Jennifer's life. "I called Brian's mother to find out about his father's doctor's visit. She told me, through tears, that the doctors were giving him one to two weeks," says Jennifer. "I had to tell Brian when he got home, but I didn't have any idea how, so I called my mother to ask her what I should say." Before Jennifer could ask, her mother announced that the doctors were worried about her liver and that she was going to get one of the most aggressive cancer treatments available, the stem cell transplant. "As soon as she told me that, Brian came home from work. I got off the phone with my mother quickly, and my legs just gave out from under me, and I fell sobbing and screaming to the floor. The whole thing was simply too much for me to process at once and was too horrible to comprehend."

The next day, she went to a psychiatrist and began taking an antidepressant, which eased her depression and anxiety. "It made it much easier for me to not constantly focus and obsess on the illness. And not obsessing made it easier to see it in perspective and not focus on her dying as much," says Jennifer. She still couldn't concentrate enough to get any good work done on her dissertation, but she functioned better in other areas of her life. "I found it much easier to do physical activities where I didn't have to think, so I took my dog for a walk for an hour and a half every day, and was doing a lot of gardening."

The following summer, her mother underwent the stem cell transplant. Because the procedure temporarily knocks out the body's immune system, her mother had to stay hospitalized for a month while her body's immunity strengthened. Jennifer had been offered a teaching position that spring at the University of Chicago, and again had to miss the first week of her mother's hospital stay, though the semester ended in time for her to make it home for the remaining three weeks of the treatment.

After her month of hospitalization, Mickey stayed with Jennifer for a week. "I scrubbed the entire house with bleach before she came because I'm not the neatest person and I was afraid she'd catch some horrid disease from the house," recalls Jennifer. Her mother, though, was antsy to get home and resume her life, and as soon as she could, she loaded herself into her car and drove back to Pennsylvania, where she is an elementary school teacher. Mickey never felt the need or the desire to slow the pace of her life or call anything off because of her cancer. She had continued teaching during her chemotherapy and had scheduled the stem cell transplant during the summer so she wouldn't have to miss any school.

Soon after the stem cell transplant, Jennifer, then twenty-eight, at the urging of her aunts, went in for a baseline mammogram, a routine exam that turned into a horror show. She went to the Johns Hopkins Breast Center, where the radiologist reads the film on the spot. The technician had to take the mammogram three times, making Jennifer nervous. "She kept redoing the left breast and I asked the technician why. She slapped this mammogram up on the light box, and there was a big white spot on my left breast exactly where my mother's tumor was. I burst into tears and started shaking and was a mess. With my mother's cancer, the worst-case scenario keeps coming true: it shouldn't have been in her liver, but it was; she shouldn't have needed a stem cell transplant, but she did. I know that I shouldn't have a tumor at my age, but I had every reason to fear that the unexpected and inexplicable had happened to me just like it did to my mother." Fortunately, the family's streak of bad luck ended here. The white blotch on the mammogram was nothing more than dense but benign breast tissue. Breast tissue can be the same density as cancerous tissue in young women, and both can show up white on a mammogram, making these films difficult to read. As women age, their breast tissue is replaced by fat tissue, which looks gray on the mammogram, so cancers are much more obvious.

Jennifer left with a clean bill of health, and though relieved about herself, she was still worried about her mother. Only six months after Mickey's stem cell transplant, while while taking the cancer prevention drug tamoxifen, her cancer recurred. Mickey began taking Taxol, a chemotherapy drug, and has been responding well. Mickey is optimistic about her future, but Jennifer still feels hopeless about her mother's prognosis to the point that she has ceased to really live her own life.

> *I'm kind of in a holding pattern. I want to be able to go take care of my mother when the time comes. I feel like there's no point in finishing my dissertation because the next natural step would be to get a job, but I don't want a job because I couldn't leave at the drop of a hat to take care of my mother. The other issue is children. I'd like to have children soon because I'd like for my mother to know my children. But if I get pregnant right now, there's no guarantee that she'd be alive in nine months, and the thought of her dying while I was pregnant or soon after is more than I could cope with. It's hard for me to think of my life moving forward without my mother.*

Even while her mother lives, Jennifer is feeling a loss, not just in the momentum of her life, but in her relationship with her mother. In some ways, their relationship is more open than it was before the cancer, but in other ways, it's more closed.

> *I can talk to her about things like when her mother died, which was something that was never discussed before. On the other hand, I don't feel like I can tell her how depressed I feel, and I've never not been able to tell her how I feel until now. I don't want her to know how much it's hurting me. I don't feel as much hope as she does, but I can't tell her that because she needs to feel hope. She's still very much fighting the cancer. So I find it hard that I can't share this with her, and feel kind of alone because of it.*

Jennifer's protective behavior is standard among mothers and daughters, although psychologists believe it's not the best approach. A mother's or daughter's thoughts and feelings may be difficult for the other to hear, but the sharing of the feelings can be a great relief to both women, and the more that can be shared, the closer the two people will be, says psychologist Roberta Hufnagel. "To be able to say, 'Mommy, I'm afraid you're going to die,' doesn't say to your mother, 'Hurry up and die.' It doesn't kill the hope. You can say these things and still say we're going to do everything we can to make you live as long as possible," says Hufnagel.

Jennifer can occasionally lift herself from her state of hopelessness and speak more rationally about her mother's prognosis, her soft voice rising with the glint of hope. When the news came out about the cancer drug Herceptin, a new type of cancer drug known as a monoclonal antibody, Jennifer went on the Internet, albeit skeptically, to find out if the drug could help her mother. Herceptin targets a protein that is overproduced by cancer cells in women who have a certain gene mutation called HER2 (human epidermal growth factor receptor 2) inhibiting tumor growth. A woman can be tested to see if her cancer has excessive amounts of the protein (about 25 to 30 percent of breast cancers do), and if it does, the drug, which was approved by the Food and Drug Administration in 1998, may be administered. Jennifer's mother tested positive for the protein, and in January 1999 she stopped taking Taxol, which had become ineffective, and began taking Herceptin. "That's made me feel a little better. I know there are people who are doing really well on the drug. At least it means there's some hope that my mother will live."

JUDY HIME-EVERSCHOR
MAGALIA, CALIFORNIA

*S*ix weeks after Judy Hime-Everschor got married in the summer of 1990, she found herself by her mother's bedside in a hospice, watching her die of breast cancer. A year and a half later, though Judy, then thirty-four, had not been diagnosed with cancer herself, she had both her breasts removed in a hotly debated procedure known as prophylactic mastectomy. When someone once said to Judy that the surgery she was considering would be deforming, she responded, "Well, death is a lot more deforming."

Judy used to think that women always survived breast cancer. That's because when her mother, Selma, was forty-four, she survived her first bout with cancer. Selma had a mastectomy, and to Judy's eleven-year-old mind, the cancer was gone and done with. After that, the family lived a relatively normal life. "I was the youngest child of four kids, and I lived at home until I was about thirty. For almost ten years, my mom and I spent the most uninterrupted time together. She was somebody I considered my best friend," explains Judy.

But during this time of seeming normalcy, Selma always lived with the fear that she would get cancer in her other breast. She went to a breast cancer specialist every six months for follow-up examinations. She felt confident that the close monitoring would detect any cancers before they became life-threatening. But it didn't. When she was sixty-one, a small lump was found in her lymph node on the same side that she had the breast cancer, and another lump was found in her other breast. The cancer had recurred. She underwent chemotherapy and radiation, but despite the treatments, more lumps turned up in her lymph nodes. She lived for another three years.

> *Up until the end, I thought my mom would live. I was in denial, based on her earlier experience with cancer and because my mother believed in positive thinking. She never admitted to me that she was going to die, and that led me to believe that she wouldn't. By stressing positive*

thinking, though, she taught me not to face reality, to the point that I didn't recognize the obvious signs. She was having a very hard time in the last six weeks, and had been admitted into the hospital. I visited her every day, and I even went over the details of her estate with her—lists of things like who owed her money, where her safe deposit box was, and even what she thought she should have on her headstone. I wrote all this down, not because I thought she was dying, but because I thought I was helping her to get it off her mind. Soon she was transferred to a hospice for respite care, which I understood to be a place she could go for four or five days to recover from her chemotherapy so my stepdad could have a break from caring for her. I was still blinded by denial. At the end of the five days, the social worker told me we could have her stay longer if we wanted, because she was 'terminal.' That was the first time I ever heard that word applied to my mother and that's when I realized she was dying. She died two days later.

"It wasn't until she died that I realized, Oh, you can die from this disease," says Judy, poking fun at her own ignorance. Judy, now forty-one, is a petite woman with a big personality, a woman who likes to regale friends with her own philosophies of life, soliloquies filled with home-grown aphorisms and funky metaphors. Judy has the energy and enthusiasm of someone who has survived a near-death experience. Only her experience was not a brush with death, but a period of her life when she was shrouded by the fear of death, a fear of breast cancer. "When a mother dies from breast cancer, it raises the level of fear in a daughter about herself, it creates grief, loss, and mourning, and all that increases fear," says UCLA psychologist David Wellisch. The fear can complicate the grieving process because you are almost grieving for your own inevitable death. When you feel you've been abandoned by your mother, through death, you feel alone and vulnerable. "This idea that I'm next in line standing at the edge of the precipice heightens this sense of vulnerability," adds Margaret Burke, a social worker for Cancer Care in New York.

I became quite certain that I was going to die young of breast cancer. Once I was in Europe on business and felt a large lump in my breast, which I knew hadn't been there three weeks before when my doctor did a breast exam. I called my doctor, came rushing home, and went straight to his office. He did a biopsy and found it was a benign cyst. It was like that for years—I'd find a lump and call the doctor in a panic. The doctor told me not to do breast self-exams because I was driving myself crazy.

Judy's fears were based on very real concerns. Not only had her mother gotten breast cancer at a young age and then later died of the disease, but two great aunts had died of breast cancer as well, which increased Judy's actual risk. Judy herself was plagued by benign cysts that kept forming in her breasts. The cysts not only are painful but can make detection of breast cancer more difficult. "I was finding more and more lumps and couldn't tell the difference between these lumps and lumps to worry about," says Judy. She also began to fear that the doctor couldn't tell the difference either, because he didn't biopsy every lump— there were just too many. "I thought, how is he deciding which ones should be biopsied and which shouldn't? It was very arbitrary, and I felt I was putting my life in his hands," says Judy.

To make matters worse, her mother's experience had diminished her confidence in the medical system. "The doctors followed my mother so closely for eighteen years, but they missed her cancer anyway," says Judy. She wonders whether the doctors who reassured her mother truly knew enough about breast cancer and had the ability to detect it, to be so reassuring. She began to question whether or not she could count on the doctors to detect a cancer early enough to save her own life. It was the lack of control and the uncertainty that Judy couldn't tolerate.

Judy went to a comprehensive cancer center for a risk assessment, where she was given her estimated lifetime risk of breast cancer based on her family history and other risk factors. Experts recommend that women with a strong family history go for risk counseling, because most women exaggerate their risk and will typically find that their real risk is substantially lower (see *Understanding Your Risk*). Judy's risk, however, was in the ballpark with what she feared—about 35 to 40 percent. Adding to Judy's problem, the cysts that were developing had increased the size of her breasts from a C cup to a DD and made them painfully tender. "My breasts became such a source of pain and worry that I didn't feel a strong attachment to them. I detached myself because I was afraid of them. They were also too large for my body, so I didn't see them as being attractive either. I was very embarrassed in many ways by them, and they didn't bring me any sexual pleasure because of all the pain," says Judy.

One day, a breast specialist mentioned to her that she might want to think about getting her breasts surgically removed. "I couldn't believe this was a decision in my life, but I realized it was one I should seriously consider," she says. Though some breast surgeons perform the procedure, most don't recommend it because it's such an aggressive strategy to lower one's risk, and it doesn't guarantee that a woman won't get cancer, because the procedure typically leaves a little breast tissue behind. However, a recent study found that it does reduce the risk of breast cancer in high risk women by 90 percent (see *Reducing Your Risk*). It also reduces a woman's fear.

"All of us have a chance of getting certain diseases, and we go through life dealing with that level of uncertainty," explains genetic counselor June Peters, who met with Judy, adding, "Judy is at the far end of the scale in terms of her need of certainty, and her experience made it intolerable for her—not knowing how to predict if she'd get it, when she'd get it, and how it would affect her life." Women who are seriously considering this option should take time to make the decision and consult with psychologists, risk counselors, surgeons, oncologists, and radiologists.

Judy did just that. She got opinions from three different breast specialists and went to a psychologist before she made the final decision to have her breasts removed.

*In therapy, I talked about my anger over the fact that
my mother's cancer was missed and that there was still no*

*cure for breast cancer, but mostly I talked about my feel-
ings about my breasts and my sexuality. Here I was deciding to do something that would be devastating to my
mother's generation and to many women. When my mother lost her breast, she said to my father, "Am I deformed
now?" But I thought, who am I? First, I'm a person, then
I'm a woman, and because I like the person so much, I
decided to try to save her.*

After Judy made the decision, she was looking for approval
from friends and family, but she found that some people reacted
negatively. "I was particularly upset when people would imply
that I might be a hypochondriac and needed to see a psychiatrist.
I was already seeing a psychologist. And besides, I thought, if I
get breast cancer, how's a psychiatrist going to help me then,"
says Judy. "My biggest fear, though, was that I might be disap-
pointing my husband because my breasts were his favorite toy.
But he seemed to understand right from the start why I would
want to remove my breasts, though he didn't want to influence
me either way."

Once she made the decision, she felt a great sense of relief
and felt that it was the right choice for her. She went to see all her
doctors again to find out exactly what the procedure entailed and
what side effects she should expect. She decided not to get breast
implants. It was around the time when the news about the dan-
gers of silicone implants was coming out. "I was not interested in
trading one problem for another," says Judy. As the day of
surgery approached, she felt a little nervous, more so about the
actual surgery with its inherent risks than about losing her
breasts. "It was so clear to me by then that this would remove so
much of my risk and my fear," says Judy.

The night before the surgery, Judy and her husband, Buddy,
had dinner at a fancy steak house and then stayed at a hotel right
next to the hospital so they could be on time for her six A.M.
surgery.

*I felt this nervousness that night, like the feeling of
starting the first day of school or a new job. There were a*

lot of questions floating around in my head. What will it be like? Will this get rid of my fear? Will I miss not having breasts? Back at the hotel, I was looking at my breasts, saying, "These won't be here anymore." It was an emotional saying good-bye for both of us, but more for my husband, because by then, I was pretty detached from them because of all the trouble they had caused me.

The next morning, Judy went in for surgery. The anesthesiologist came and spoke to her, and she was taken into a room for the IV. "That's when Buddy and I had to separate, and that was really scary for me. All of a sudden I was afraid I would never see him again," says Judy. The doctor came in and took a few pictures of her breasts. "I remember wanting to make some joke about how he could sell them, but I didn't," she recalls.

The surgery was four hours long. When the surgeon removed her breasts, he was surprised at how packed they were with cysts. He biopsied about fifteen from each breast, and they were all benign. "When I woke up, I didn't feel anything, but I looked down. I had a gown on and saw that I was flat chested. The first thing I said to Buddy was, 'It's over,' and I was referring not to the surgery but to the fear."

Judy was in the hospital for three days and suffered little pain. Before she could leave, her doctor had to remove her bandages. It wasn't by any means the moment of reckoning; she wasn't waiting with anticipation to see what she looked like. "I think I was pushing away any emotions at the time," says Judy. "I just kept saying to myself, I don't have to worry any more." When he removed the bandages, she was more focused on the details, like how thin the scar was, not on the overall picture. She was thinking of the benefits. She could stand up straight for the first time; her body looked more in proportion now. Later on, she found that clothes looked better on her and that for the first time in many years, she could walk around braless and feel a cool breeze against her chest.

The doctor told Judy that she should wait until she healed to show her husband. When she got home, Buddy asked her how it looked. "I said, 'It looks okay.' He said, 'Can I see it?' I said, 'The doctor says you probably shouldn't. Do you want to?' He said 'Sure,' so I showed him and he said, 'Wow, the scar is so thin.' He wasn't repulsed. He treated it as if I had my appendix out," says Judy. As time passed, she adds, "He did say he misses my breasts, but that he has me, and that's more important to him."

I don't see my life without breasts as a tragedy. My mother died this horrible death. I spent a lot of time with her during the last stages, and it was very frightening. In a matter of months, she went from being a strong woman to someone who couldn't make it across the room without having to stop to rest. And she spent eighteen years of her life fearing the disease that ultimately killed her. That is a tragedy. I didn't want to live that way or die that way. The major effect the surgery has had on my life is that I don't live with the fear anymore. The quality of our life is totally different now because I don't think about cancer. We used to talk about my breasts all the time.

Since the procedure, Judy's life has taken a new course. She went to graduate school and is pursuing her license as a marriage, family, and child counselor. Among the women she counsels are those considering prophylactic mastectomy. Judy continued to see a therapist herself after her surgery to deal with the feelings of grief for her mother, which she had suppressed. After her mother's death, Judy had escaped into work and dealing with her mother's estate. "I also suppressed my pain by telling myself I was relieved she had died so that she wouldn't have to suffer anymore," says Judy. But she had lost her mother, her best friend, and the one person in her life who would unconditionally shower her with praise and love. Now, Judy has another thing to grieve: her breasts. "It was a loss. More than anything, I would have liked to have had nice normal breasts like everyone else—breasts that bring them sexual pleasure. I felt cheated. I would have liked to have had safe breasts," says Judy.

When I used to tell my mother I found another lump, she would always say, "Oh, I'm so sorry." She seemed to feel this deep sense of pain that she had passed it on to me. But I have everything—a great life, a wonderful husband. And I just didn't want to throw it all away.

8

IN OUR MOTHERS'
VOICES

"I don't want my daughter to have to go through what I went through."

Mickey D'Urso, 48

An odd phenomenon recurred in the office of psychologist David Wellisch at the University of California at Los Angeles while he was interviewing women who had breast cancer. When the conversation would lead to a particular subject, the women became extremely anxious, so anxious that they were unable to remain seated in their chairs. The subject was their daughters.

It's hard to imagine that a woman diagnosed with a life-threatening illness, who's running around in a panic, trying to absorb all the new information, making choices about her body and her life, and alternately being run down by the side effects of radiation and chemotherapy, would have any emotional energy left to worry about her children. Yet Wellisch found, and I've learned from my own interviews with women, that mothers, even when very sick, are still mothers. As much as they fear for themselves, they worry about their children.

Cynthia, a daughter, told this poignant story of her mother in the final stages of her illness. The doctors had ordered an X ray of her mother's esophagus, and her mother was strapped onto a machine, which rotated her horizontally.

She was very ill. Her stomach was bloated, her body was distorted, she was weak, and they wanted me to stay with her to hold her hand during the X ray because it was so scary. But my mother said, "No, Cindy, you go behind the glass." She said to the technician, "This is my daughter; she's going to have kids. She shouldn't stay in here." As sick as my mother was, three weeks from dying, she was worrying that her daughter would be exposed to X rays. She was as protective of us in her death as she was in her life.

Every woman who is diagnosed with breast cancer will handle it differently. Every woman has her own way of coping with the disease and of dealing with her children. But there are commonalities in their experiences, their thoughts, and their feelings, especially when it comes to their feelings about their children. For daughters, understanding the mother's perspective may help deal with some of the mixed signals and conflicting emotions witnessed throughout diagnosis, treatment, and recovery.

When a woman is diagnosed with breast cancer, she is usually knocked off her feet by competing gusts of emotions—disbelief, denial, panic, fear, anger, sadness, loneliness, and grief for her body and her life. It happens suddenly. One day she feels healthy and is thinking about the mundane details of life; the next day, she still feels healthy but is now thinking of surgery, disfigurement, chemotherapy, and death. She quickly has to find her footing, because there's usually a sense of urgency, to get treated, to extricate the cancer. She needs to think clearly, to absorb what seems like tomes of information about breast cancer. She has to face her treatment options, to make life-and-death decisions, lumpectomy vs. mastectomy, reconstruction, chemotherapy, and radiation. She vacillates between fearing and coping, sadness and hope. Indeed, an estimated 25 percent of women show signs of depression for one year after diagnosis, according to University of Washington's Frances Marcus Lewis.

But as she is fearing for her own life, she is also worrying about how her children will manage without her, even if her absence is just temporary. A mother with toddlers or school-age

children immediately worries about what she should do with
the children while she's sick and who will take care of them,
says Sandra Haber, PhD, a psychologist who counsels women
with breast cancer. If the children are older, her fears might focus
on a future that she won't be part of. She might be saddened
that she may not be there to see her daughter's wedding or her
grandchildren.

"I had a five-year-old and six-year-old when I was diagnosed," says Mary, a forty-two-year-old nurse from California
whose mother also had breast cancer. "Since my own mother had
died young, I was terrified of leaving them alone. All I could
think about was, if something happens to me, what would happen to them. That was my total focus. I could feel myself getting
depressed, and I remember thinking, I'm not dead yet, I have to
begin to live in every moment."

As things settle down, to the degree that they do, and
women have a chance to absorb the implications of their illness
and the day-to-day effects of treatment, other issues begin to
arise, many of which go to the heart of what it means to be a
mother, to be the protector of your children, the nurturer, the
healer, and in our culture, to be supermom. These roles, of
course, are often compromised by cancer. A mother may not be
able to be the nurturer she was, and in fact she may feel like she
has brought hardship on the family rather than alleviating her
family's pain and suffering.

In her study, Lewis found that mothers with breast cancer
who had school-age children were distressed by their own limitations. Some said they felt too sick or tired to help their children,
too worried about their own survival, or too depleted emotionally to be the nurturer. It is difficult for mothers to relinquish some
of their motherly roles, even while they are sick. "Not being able
to mother their children has completely decimated some
women," adds Haber. "There's a feeling of failing their own
child. There's a terrible loss for mothers, mixed with a lot of
worry, which can lead to anxiety or depression or even feelings of
resentment."

They feel even worse about it when there is any kind of
role reversal with their daughters, as Sandy, a mother of two,

experienced when her daughter Jill (see *Mothering Mom*) began caring for her and taking over the household.

"My daughter, who was nineteen when I was diagnosed, was doing most of the housework," says Sandy. "I felt so bad that the pressure was on her. I wanted to be able to do the laundry, to cook, to shop; that's what I was supposed to be doing. I've always been very nurturing. I wanted everything to be good for my family. I've learned I can't do that anymore. But I have a hard time giving in and saying okay, I'm tired. I try to be nurturing in other ways now that don't require a physical outlay of energy. Just by talking more and being supportive in whatever ways I can. Once I finish the radiation, maybe I'll be able to do as much as I used to, but I can't do that anymore now."

The myth of the supermom only adds to the inadequacy women feel. "I'm the sort of person who wants to be in control and do everything and take care of everyone's needs," says Noella, who has four grown daughters and has recently immigrated to the United States from India. "My daughters are trying to give me permission to say I don't have to be that way. They say they're here to take over, to help, but it's hard to let go."

"Nurturing one's children is so central to a mother," adds psychologist Evelyn Bassoff, "and when she's no longer able to do that, she can suffer a profound feeling of loss." But a mother who can take the pressure off herself will be able to have more give-and-take in her relationships with her children. "The mother has to change from being the nurturer and giver to becoming the receiver, and receiving in a gracious way. Some women feel so guilty and unused to this role of receiving attention that they act irritable and annoyed," says Bassoff.

Likewise, mothers are often cautious about overburdening their daughters emotionally. Mothers try not to reveal just how bad they feel, physically or emotionally.

"My feeling was that I didn't want my daughters to be hurting, and I knew how much they were," says Lola, a retired mother of three daughters in their late thirties and forties. "I do try to protect them because they're my children, and I want to spare them as much pain as I can. We've always tried not to burden one another. I'm sure they've tried to shield me, too."

Adds Mickey, whose daughter Jennifer, a twenty-nine-year-old, is her only child (see *Depression and Fear*), "I probably would have lied to my daughter about the metastasis had she not come with me to the doctor to get the results of the baseline liver scan, bone scan, and chest X ray. She insisted on going, and she heard that there was something wrong with my liver. That set the tone for honesty from the outset. I'm glad that it did. I realize now that it's not fair to treat other people who are adults, who are concerned, as patronizingly as that."

Indeed, protecting a daughter from the truth can do more damage than good. "In my experience, whenever people are honest with each other, though it's painful during the conversation and difficult things are brought up, as they go through the process, there's a real sense of relief," says Bassoff. "When you are truly honest with somebody, there is intimacy." This intimacy can lead to an even deeper bond and greater understanding between mothers and daughters. Without honesty, daughters complain of feeling helpless or useless in the face of their mother's illness. They didn't know how their mother felt, so they were unable to help ease her emotional concerns or her physical discomfort.

But there's a limit to what mothers will tell, a boundary between mother and daughter that remains. "Mothers should be careful not to lay all their anxieties on their children. A child is not a friend and a child is not a therapist," says Haber. If a mother goes on and on about her fear of dying, it may echo a daughter's own fears and serve to increase her level of insecurity and anxiety. Some mothers will reserve these more difficult feelings for their friends and support groups.

Mothers are also keenly aware of their daughters' futures. They know that because breast cancer can be hereditary, their own diagnosis nudges their daughters over the line and into the high-risk group. Some women feel guilty that they are passing down this genetic legacy to their daughters, as if they could have done something in their life to cause or to prevent the mutation. They know that it is not rational—that if the gene mutation exists in their family, it is not their fault, but they still feel somehow responsible.

"I knew my children were going to be so terribly upset, so it was really difficult to tell them about my cancer," says Lola. "I felt that in some way I had failed them by getting cancer. I had been so healthy and strong. We've always had this belief that our genes are wonderful."

Adds Karen, founder of the Sisters Network, a national support group for African American women who have breast cancer, "Logically, I know I shouldn't feel guilty, but emotionally, I know I have put an extra burden and emotional strain on my daughter. I didn't grow up having to worry about cancer. The younger generation has a lot more to deal with. Now she has the burden of concern for her own self." (See *Making a Difference*.)

Whether they feel guilty or not, most mothers are deeply saddened for their daughters. One evening, nine-year-old Anna, with curly red hair, blue eyes, and cappuccino skin, looked up at her mother, Alicia, who was sick from chemotherapy, and asked, "When I get breast cancer, will you take care of me like Grandma takes care of you?" It nearly broke her mother's heart. She thought, Why should Anna, still young enough to play with dolls, have to be so cognizant of a mortal disease and already so certain of her own morbid fate?

Says Mickey, "I know that my daughter is worried for herself. You'd have to be crazy to be third generation and not be. Fortunately, she seems to take after her father's side of the family in personality and appearance. It would be a hell of a thing if the one thing she gets from me is this genetic defect. I don't feel guilty about it, because I can't control it. I just feel sick about it and scared. I don't want her to have to go through what I went through, and I don't want her to have to live with the specter of it."

The fear springs from two sources. Mothers worry about their daughters getting breast cancer and having to endure the emotional and physical hardship of the disease. They also feel bad that their daughters now have to live with the fear, that their lives can no longer be as carefree as they had been before cancer. They are saddened to see in their daughters the loss of innocence, the loss of that sense of invulnerability that young people have.

"We've never had a history of breast cancer. So it was awful for me to be the one introducing it to my whole family," says Noella, adding, "They have all told their gynecologists and doctors they have this history. I feel very upset about this."

Some mothers, though, are truly hopeful about their daughters' futures, just as they were optimistic about their own battles with cancer. Usually, the women who fared well during treatment and became survivors are the most optimistic about their daughters' fate. They believe that medical science is close to finding an acceptable cure or prevention, and will do so before their daughters are diagnosed. "To me, it doesn't matter if my daughter gets breast cancer or not," says Alicia, a second generation survivor. "It's that she is given enough education, real life experiences, resources, and enough care that she can work through it. Just as long as she has all the knowledge, I think she'll be okay." Other mothers can't even talk about the prospect of their daughters getting cancer without breaking into tears.

9

MAKING A
DIFFERENCE

"She would have been proud that I'm doing something to help other people. I'm just sorry I couldn't have done more to help her."

Marcia Presky, 43

CALEEN BURTON-ALLEN
HOUSTON, TEXAS

Caleen Burton-Allen's great-great aunt died without anyone ever knowing she had breast cancer. "It didn't come out until they were dressing her body for the funeral and found that she had a double mastectomy," says Caleen, a thirty-four-year-old mother of two. "That's sad. She went to her grave with that secret." Then, years later, her great aunt died of breast cancer, and the cause of her death was also not discussed.

Keeping cancer a secret was part of the culture of her family, says Caleen, and it's typical of many African American families like her own. "It's always been a common understanding in the black community that you don't talk about certain things. The C word was one of the things you didn't discuss, and you definitely didn't discuss it with people outside your family," says Caleen. Many African Americans have viewed cancer as a disgrace, she says, as if it means something is wrong with their family, so they keep it to themselves.

But when Caleen's own mother, Karen, was diagnosed with breast cancer in October 1993 at the age of fifty, she couldn't subscribe to this unhealthy tradition. "Despite my upbringing, for some reason I've always been open about most everything," says Karen, who is a survivor. "The question never entered my mind not to speak out about breast cancer in my family, especially once I learned that your family history is very important. It was more a matter of how long it would take for my family to accept the conversation."

Breaking the silence was an admirable but not easy goal. "When my mother started getting out there and telling family members she had breast cancer, my grandmother would call her and say, 'Why are you talking about it? We know you have breast cancer; you don't have to broadcast it,'" recalls Caleen, who is a freelance journalist and the public relations manager for the Port of Houston Authority. The older generation were resistant, but the younger generation, Caleen's generation, were grateful. Her mother received calls from cousins and nieces thanking her for finally bringing cancer out of the family closet. Actually, some thanks are owed to Caleen. When Karen was diagnosed six years ago, she was so shocked by the news that she went into denial. For several weeks, she didn't tell anyone, not her husband nor Caleen, her only child. "I was surprised my mother shut down quite as much as she did," says Caleen. "She had been getting mammograms and had been well informed and was taking the right precautions. But when she was diagnosed, she couldn't think. She couldn't think of what the logical next step would be, what her options were, what surgery she should have. She just was not dealing with it and was saying things like 'I'll put it off for a little while.'"

Once her mother revealed the truth, Caleen took command of the situation. "I went into my journalist mode and began researching treatments—the hospitals in her area, the doctors," says Caleen. She sent her mother articles and books on breast cancer, trying to arm her with enough information on all her options for her to make smart choices. "My mom wanted to postpone making any decisions, partly because we were planning my wedding, which was only one month away, but I said to her,

'The doctors say you need to do it now. That's when we're going to do it, and if that means putting everything else on hold, then so be it. Your health is first and foremost.'"

With her intelligent and very persuasive daughter urging her to face her illness, Karen didn't have much choice but to snap out of her own inertia. Once mobilized, she went completely in the other direction. "When my mother did finally come to terms with her breast cancer, there was no stopping her. She tried to discuss this disease with people, to find out what services were available to her, and to get all the information she could about breast cancer and her treatment options," says Caleen. Adds her mother, "I wanted to know how this was going to affect my life. I started looking for answers, but I had a hard time finding them. I found that not only was my own family not talking about cancer, but neither were my personal friends and women I'd meet in social situations—nobody wanted to talk about it. So I started seeking out black women who were breast cancer survivors, which wasn't easy."

After doing research, Karen decided to have a lumpectomy, followed by chemotherapy and radiation. A month or two into her chemotherapy treatment, Karen cofounded a breast cancer support group for African Americans in Los Angeles, where she lived. At the same time, she pushed ahead with planning Caleen's wedding, which was to be held in Los Angeles. "I thought the wedding could wait, that we should call it off, but she felt that we should continue as we had planned," says Caleen. The wedding pushed her mother to her physical limits, but at the same time, it was a mental antidote to the cancer, as it was an exciting and time-consuming distraction from the disease and the side effects of the treatments. "She was really incredible. She showed me how much somebody could do when they put their mind to it," says Caleen.

Eight months later, in July 1994, Karen moved to Houston and decided to launch a national support group organization— the Sisters Network, Inc. In a little over four years, the network has grown to eighteen chapters nationwide. Karen's main goal is to educate women about the appropriate services and treatment standards. "There are racial biases that hinder the quality of life of black women with cancer, such as not being offered certain treatments or being asked to come back in six months for follow-up screenings," says Karen. Indeed, for various reasons, including problems with their access to health care, African American women are two to three times less likely to get mammograms than white women and have a lower chance of surviving the disease. There are also inequalities in the services provided to survivors. "I found that several services that were available for white women weren't available for African Americans, like free wigs or appropriate shades of makeup," says Karen.

"My mom's a gung-ho kind of person and I'm not surprised she founded the Sisters Network, Inc., and it's filling the void for the African American community," says Caleen. For Karen, who had always taken jobs in her husbands' businesses, the network became her first significant enterprise, the first passionate endeavor. Karen spends most of her waking hours speaking with women with breast cancer from around the country, women who call her with their fears of cancer and their frustrations with their medical care. The phone wakes her up early in the morning and puts her to bed late at night.

But while Karen has eased her fear and sadness through her efforts to help others, Caleen hasn't been as successful in handling her own fears on the prospect of losing her mother.

> *I internalized a lot of it. It's my personality to go seek within and try to resolve my issues. But that can be lonely. I'm an only child and I was never the type to yearn for brothers and sisters. But this was the first time I had ever wished I had a brother or sister. A parent's illness is a heavy weight to carry by yourself. When I first found out, I didn't know who to call; there was no one. Friends can only go to a certain point, but a sibling has as much of an interest in it as you do. There really wasn't anyone to talk to who was going through what I was. I'm an emotional person, but I tried to be as strong as I could be for my mother. It was tough and it was something I was consumed with every single day while it was happening. Suddenly, it seemed like everywhere I turned, there was*

breast cancer. It was in my face constantly, with public service announcements, news reports, and then always hearing about breast cancer from my mom's organization.

Caleen has followed in her mother's advocacy footsteps, helping her with the Sisters Network by handling the public relations, doing fund raising, and serving on the board, but she does it more to help her mother than for any cathartic release she gets from it. In fact, it all becomes a bit much for her at times. "One night, my mother called me and started to update me on the organization, and I said, 'Can we just talk, but not about breast cancer and not about the organization? Sometimes, I'd just like you to be my mother.' Normally, I let her go on about it, but that day I had had enough," recalls Caleen. With her mother's constant talk about breast cancer, it was impossible for Caleen to push her fears to the back of her mind. "I'm not consumed by cancer, but out of seven days a week, it comes up in my mind about four or five times," says Caleen. According to research by the Strang Cancer Prevention Center's Kathryn Kash, daughters are frequently plagued with thoughts about breast cancer. But being able to forget about cancer in their day-to-day life is an important coping tactic. Otherwise, they end up preoccupied with their fears, and their fears begin to escalate, as was the case with Caleen.

After I had my first daughter, in October 1994, I found a lump and that scared the crap out of me. All my risks were running through my mind—my mother had breast cancer, I just had a baby, which puts you at a higher risk of cancer if you have your first after thirty, and I hadn't had a mammogram yet. The funny thing was that despite all I knew about breast cancer, I did exactly what my mother did when she had a lump. I went into denial. I didn't say anything to my mother for about four or five days. I didn't say anything to anyone, not even my husband. I was petrified to think that I might have cancer. I was thinking, I have a brand new baby; what if I die? I was in a daze, kind of talking myself out of it, saying, oh, you really didn't find anything, it's nothing.

Here she was, armed with even more information than her mother had when she was diagnosed, and reacting the same exact way. "It's very scary," says Caleen, who suddenly understood why women avoid cancer screening. Finally, Caleen told her mother, who immediately brought Caleen to her surgeon. She had a mammogram, and a breast specialist did a needle biopsy of the lump, which turned out to be a clogged milk duct.

Aside from worrying about herself, Caleen still fears that she will lose her mother. "My mother is busy worrying about everyone else in her network, and I'm worrying about her," says Caleen. "Whenever she's not feeling well, I start thinking the worst. Every time she goes and has her different routine tests, brings it to the front burner and incites that fear in me again. When the tests come back clean, I breathe a little easier, but I know that tests don't guarantee anything."

On the other side of fear is a gratefulness for life. It is impossible for Caleen to take her mother for granted after going through this.

> *Breast cancer put everything into perspective in my life. After I got married, my mother moved here to Houston from LA. I think she moved to be with me and my girls. It meant a lot to have her here when I had my daughters and for her to have a relationship with them. She tries to expose them to all kinds of experiences, as she did with me when I was growing up. I'm really proud of my mother and what she's done with the Sisters Network. She's a wonderful person. It's really important to me that my kids know my mother well.*

MARCIA PRESKY
NEW YORK, NEW YORK

On a spring day in 1995, Marcia Presky, a thirty-nine-year-old New Yorker, stood in front of an audience of Czech women in a stuffy university classroom in Prague and talked about her mother's breast cancer and her mother's death. The women, listening intensely through an interpreter, all had had breast cancer. Some were recently diagnosed, some were twenty-five-year survivors, and many of them had daughters of their own. None of them, however, had ever heard anyone speak so openly about their experiences with this illness. Marcia told them how shocked and saddened she felt when her mother was diagnosed, how angry she felt toward certain callous doctors, and how she feels persistent grief over her mother's death. Above all, she told them about her biggest regret—she and her mother were never able to open up to each other, not even during her mother's illness.

The silence that came between mother and daughter is what brought Marcia all the way to the Czech Republic and placed her in front of these women. Not long after her own mother's death in 1991, Marcia set out on a mission to encourage women with cancer to be open with their family and friends. With hindsight, she believes the burden of the illness should not be carried alone. Marcia, now forty-three, organized the weeklong workshop in Prague and brought with her a delegation of two American breast cancer survivors from SHARE, a self-help support group in New York City for women with breast or ovarian cancer. Before this, she had been working on a project in the Czech Republic for her job in international development, and while there, she recognized that Czech women were far behind Americans in feminist and women's health issues. "I thought these SHARE women have been through the women's movement, they've been through the cancer experience, wouldn't it be great for them to work with women over there," says Marcia.

Marcia would much rather talk about Prague or SHARE or anything but her own experience of her mother's breast cancer. She has many regrets. But seated stiffly in her apartment in Greenwich Village, she reluctantly opens up as she searches for the memories. Marcia was twenty-three years old when she returned from a two-week vacation in Peru to learn that her mother had found a lump in her breast and was going to have it biopsied. That was back in 1978, in the days when a woman would go in for a biopsy and if the lump was malignant, the surgeon would perform a mastectomy without consulting the woman or her family. There were no options. "I remember waiting at the hospital with my father. We really didn't talk about stuff that much, but I knew he was thinking that the surgery was taking a long time and that meant it's probably cancer. He was visibly shaken up, and he was right," recalls Marcia.

When the surgeon came out to deliver the news, Marcia and her father were already stricken with grief. Marcia recalls that the surgeon, who worked at a leading cancer center in New York City, told them that it was malignant and then said to Marcia, "Don't worry. Your mother is healthy now." These words were tough to absorb after having just heard the word *malignant*. "It was hard to believe him, especially since we hadn't gotten the tests back about the lymph nodes, but I thought, he's a big surgeon, so he would know, and I took some kind of solace in his prognosis." It was all Marcia had to grasp onto at the time.

It turned out that the surgeon was wrong, that her mother was not healthy, and that she had several lymph nodes that were malignant, a sign that the disease was more advanced. The mastectomy was followed by a six-month course of chemotherapy. "My mother came home and we didn't really talk about the operation or the chemo. Looking back, I wish we could have talked about it—I could have helped her and she could have helped me," explains Marcia. "We talked, but about external things like current events or issues, just not about feelings."

After the chemotherapy, Marcia's mother, Esther, went back to her normal life, acting as if nothing had happened. "She never showed me the mastectomy scar. I remember seeing it once in the dressing room of a department store. I thought, it's not very attractive, but then again, it's not the worst thing in the world either. I wasn't horrified. I remember wondering how I would deal with something like this," says Marcia. But she kept her poker face, incapable of expressing any of these thoughts or showing any reaction to her mother.

Three years after Esther passed the five-year mark, when the risk of recurrence drops dramatically, she broke a rib, for no obvious cause. She underwent a series of tests, which revealed that the cancer had metastasized to her bones. She immediately began receiving hormonal treatments, drugs similar to tamoxifen, which block estrogen from attaching to the cancerous cells in order to inhibit their growth. She continued with various hormonal drugs for five years. They were long, anxiety-ridden years, filled with the emotional highs and lows that come with the ever-changing news, the success of one treatment, the failure of another, remission and recurrence, and for Esther, the five years finally ended in death.

"After the cancer had metastasized, I began thinking about and dealing with her cancer on a day-to-day basis, wondering what the next blood test would show and whether the treatment was still working," says Marcia. It was stressful for Marcia because she could not tell how her mother was handling the disease or how sick she was feeling. "Because we really didn't openly communicate, I was always fearing the worst." When Esther would return from a doctor's visit, she would relate the medical details to Marcia but nothing else. It was a very matter-of-fact report, minus emotions. Marcia would say "Gee, that's great" if everything looked good. If it didn't, she wouldn't say anything. She felt she had to react in silence and appear expressionless. "It worked for me in some respects in that I didn't have to open up and tell her my feelings. But another part of me would have liked to have been there at a different level for both my parents. What was most difficult for me was feeling powerless to help in any way and too afraid to ask what was going on inside. Here was my mother who was very sick, and I didn't know what the progression of the disease would be, and I didn't know how to support her through it." The situation left Marcia with a low level depression and a constant preoccupation with her mother's disease.

Since Esther's death, Marcia has moments when she feels angry at her mother, a distressing emotion that often comes with the baggage of guilt and shame, despite how common it is among the bereaved. She is angry that her mother didn't communicate and angry at herself for not being able to change their unhealthy patterns. "If the mother didn't want to talk and the daughter feels that she never got to say things, it can lead to anger, frustration, guilt, and great sadness in the daughter," explains Cancer Care's Patricia Spicer.

Thinking back, Marcia was surprised that the crises of her mother's cancer didn't open up everyone as much as she had hoped. In fiction and in the movies, illness is typically portrayed as a catalyst for dramatic change. The reality for some families is that even life-threatening illness doesn't necessarily change the dynamics between mothers and daughters. Indeed, often it just emphasizes good relationships and exacerbates bad ones. "You are who you are, and you're even more who you are when you're sick," says New York City psychologist Allison Ross. The fantasy that illness will heal poor relationships between mothers and daughters could be dangerous because it sets the daughter up for disappointment when nothing changes, she adds.

Marcia also wished she had had some support of her own. She kept her sadness and her fears to herself, repressing them, not revealing them to anyone, not her family nor her friends. Marcia did manage to put herself into therapy, which became her one outlet for her emotions. Toward the end of her mother's life, the psychologist helped Marcia to try to bond with her mother. "The therapy gave me tools and ways to talk with my mother that were more comfortable for her," says Marcia. "I'd spend time with her in more intimate ways, doing physical things like massaging her feet, things that she wouldn't have allowed me to do in the past. So by the end, we had a certain relationship and understanding that was fairly comfortable. But there was unfinished business that I wished we had taken care of."

For Marcia, taking action was one way she could overcome her unresolved feelings, so she decided to join the SHARE advocacy committee. "I wanted to become involved in the fight for a cure for the disease and for better care for women coping with the illness," says Marcia. Volunteering for a breast cancer organization is the kind of work that can give a daughter's own suffering meaning, by sharing her experience to benefit others and by passing on something from her and from her mother, explains genetic counselor June Peters.

At SHARE, Marcia finally met women she was able to talk to and who openly shared their feelings with her. "I began to get from them what I wasn't able to get from my mother, which is not the same, but it provided an outlet for me to deal with some of the feelings I wasn't able to face with my mother. I was hesitant at first to talk with them because my mother's outcome wasn't a good one and I didn't want to scare them. But I soon realized that these women understood only too well that some women die from breast cancer, and they were able to listen to me anyway." Marcia experienced the bond among survivors, the connection formed by that unspoken sense of knowing, a simple nod that communicates complete empathy. The people at SHARE believe that you can contribute to your own healing by helping others, which was the road to wellness that Marcia wanted to take.

I had the idea that the Czech women would benefit from meeting the SHARE women in learning how to develop self-help activities, how to educate themselves, and how to do advocacy work. I thought we could use breast cancer education to empower women in all different aspects of their lives. When you teach a woman to talk to her doctor about what she needs, you're teaching her how to talk to other authority figures about what she needs.

She formed a collaboration between SHARE and her employer, the American Jewish Joint Distribution Committee, and organized three week-long workshops, which together sowed the seeds of a breast cancer advocacy movement there. The workshops had a liberating effect on the Czech women. Never had the breast cancer experience been acknowledged before for these women. They were accustomed to hiding, hiding their bodies and hiding their personal struggles.

In the Czech Republic, it went like this: You have cancer, you get your breast cut off, that's the end. The family wanted to think everything was fine. Some women didn't tell their husbands that they were ill until after the surgery. Some women said they were diagnosed and treated fifteen years ago, but this was the first time they were talking about it. During the workshop, there was such incredible bonding among these women because their experiences had been validated for the first time. There was a lot of hugging and crying and laughing. They had that real heartfelt appreciation, that we came all the way there from America to talk with them.

For Marcia, the experience was both difficult and gratifying. "Speaking about my experience is hard; it is never easy talking about the period when my mother was very sick and dying; it's still very emotionally charged. I do it because it is gratifying to know that in my way, I am helping other women and helping to increase resources to find the cure," says Marcia.

The workshops were also a success for women's issues in the Czech Republic. They introduced the idea of self-help and support groups to women there and spurred a series of action plans to provide new services and better care, including a national resource and information database, educational programs, and better mammography equipment. The Prague women even started a petition drive, writing down their names and ID numbers, an exercise in freedom of speech that ran counter to their cultural upbringing and was unheard of during the communist era in which they were raised. They presented the petition to the Ministry. "That was the epitome of success, empowering these women to put themselves out there, put their names down, and give that to the government," says Marcia. The most visible result from her workshops, however, was the recent announcement by the first lady of the Czech Republic that she was designating breast cancer as her number one cause. After seeing the success in Prague, Marcia launched a similar program in Israel, which quite amazingly is bringing together secular women, ultra-Orthodox Jews, and Arab women on the issue of breast cancer.

Marcia's success is a testament to how much power a mother can have even in, or perhaps especially in, her death.

> *I couldn't get what I needed from my own mother, but here I am helping a million other adults. I got into this to help in ways that I couldn't help with my own family. I kind of feel I did this in honor of my mother. She would have been proud that I'm doing something to help other people. I'm just sorry I couldn't have done more to help her.*

10

CHANGE FROM WITHIN

"What is the point of this unless you can come out of it having grown, or having learned, or being available for someone else who is going through a similar situation?"

Cynthia Cohen, 31

CYNTHIA COHEN
NEW YORK, NEW YORK

Having stopped to get gas while running errands on a sunny morning in Florida, Cynthia Cohen and her father came upon what Cynthia describes as "two gorgeous blond hippie guys" who were going out to surf. "I was twenty-five, and I remember thinking, I am not going to hang out with these guys. I am not going to be carefree. Right now, my responsibility is to be with my mother who is dying," says Cynthia, now thirty-one. "Here were these two hot-looking guys going off to the beach, and I was going to the hospital."

In that moment, she realized that there had been a shift inside her. In the month that she had been watching her mother die of breast cancer, Cynthia, a commodities broker on Wall Street, had begun to grow up and become a more caring, spiritual person.

It began on the day after her brother's twenty-fifth birthday, in November 1993. Cynthia, who has a slender build, fair wispy hair, and fine features, was relaxing in her Upper West Side apartment in New York City when her mother, Dale, called from Florida.

"It's come back," said Dale.

Cynthia knew instantly what "it" was, even though more than five years had passed since her mother was first diagnosed and treated for breast cancer. Since then, Cynthia and her brother had always been nervous about a recurrence, dreading their mother's follow-up exams and her mammograms and checking in regularly with her to make sure she had no unusual symptoms. They were especially protective of their mother because their parents had divorced many years ago, and she had not remarried. At the five-year mark, Cynthia and her brother had breathed a collective sigh of relief. Just when Cynthia had begun to put cancer behind her, the call came, and it came with absolutely the worst prognosis. "Even when she told me, I thought all right, we have time, we can do a million things to fight this," recalls Cynthia. It turns out that Dale's cancer was in its final stage. The next day, her mother was so ill that she admitted herself to the hospital.

What Cynthia soon learned shocked her. Dale had a recurrence two years earlier (within the five-year window) but decided to keep it a secret from her children until the last possible moment. She also decided that she couldn't go through chemotherapy again and essentially chose not to treat her cancer. "The fact that she didn't tell me was extraordinary. We were very, very close. There were no secrets. My mother used to talk to me about the minutiae of life, like what I had for breakfast. For her to keep that from me was almost mind boggling. We used to ask her all the time, 'Mom, is everything okay?' when she had mammograms and doctor's visits. She'd say 'Everything is fine. Don't worry about me.' She basically lied to us," says Cynthia, without a hint of anger in her voice. Though Cynthia would have liked to have had more time with her mother, she doesn't feel angry at her for withholding the truth.

I think she made that decision because my brother and I had both recently graduated from college and she didn't want her illness be the thing in our lives that was most prevalent. She didn't want us to be burdened with the sadness or the responsibility of her illness. She wanted us to lead our lives. She wanted to protect her children.

That night, Cynthia called her brother and the two stayed up and cried and planned and talked all evening. Cynthia flew down to Florida the next day; her brother followed the day after. The last time Cynthia had seen her mother, only three weeks earlier when her mother was in New York City for a visit, she looked as vivacious as she always had. Her mother was a charismatic and gregarious woman, and there was no sign that these qualities were fading. But the woman Cynthia found when she entered the hospital room was thin, weak, and wan. As soon as she saw how ill her mother was, she called her office and asked for a leave of absence. She and her brother often stood watch by her until she died exactly a month later.

> *It was a wonderful month we spent together in many ways. My brother and I were very (united) with her; we didn't leave her side. We were very involved in every decision. I would go with her for every test and we were there day and night except to sleep. Because my parents were divorced, it was really just the three of us. It was a time when we were all together. It was a very loving time. We would talk to her and comfort her. She didn't talk to us much about the illness, even when she was dying. I think she was so sad she was dying and didn't want to face it. We used to get on the bed, and we would snuggle with her, my brother too; we would comb her hair or help her put on her makeup. Mostly, I remember these physical moments.*

But it wasn't just companionship that Cynthia provided. She took on a tremendous amount of responsibility. Cynthia's father had flown down to Florida because he wanted to say his good-byes to his ex-wife and also to help his children sort out the financial issues and arrange for the funeral. "If you strip away the emotional aspect of dealing with your mother who is so ill and who you just want to protect from everything," says Cynthia, "there's also an enormous organizational aspect of caregiving. Working on Wall Street, I'm rarely daunted by things, but this was very stressful for me."

Cynthia's mother asked her children to bring her home to die, a feat that is complicated to orchestrate. Having their mother die at home put more pressure on Cynthia and her brother, because they had to assume more responsibility in making sure she was well taken care of and her pain was being treated. They had long lists of details to arrange before they could take their mother out of the hospital. "We brought her home to my grandmom's because we were all staying in her apartment together. She was so cute in the ambulance; she was very sick, but she was happy to be out of the hospital," says Cynthia. They hired a twenty-four-hour nurse and a hospice nurse, who came to the house every day to monitor her mother and give her pain medication. At one point, Cynthia and her brother decided to take a two-day break and flew back to New York City because they didn't want to feel as though they were on a death watch.

> *I remember when I returned, I came in and she was in a lot of pain. The nurses hadn't given her enough morphine, so I immediately went into the kitchen and ground up some morphine the way the doctors had told me to. I had to put all my needs aside because I didn't want her to be in pain. That was my overriding concern. I remember feeling like this was really a shift in my life. My mother had been the one who fed me soup when I was sick. Now I was the one taking care of her and doing things that were very hard. Here I was giving my mother morphine.*

It was another shift. Cynthia had stepped into the mother's role and given up the daughter's, and in so doing, she left behind the neediness and dependence of youth. A few days later, with Cynthia and her brother at their mother's side, holding her, loving her, and reassuring her, she let go of life.

> *During the time that she was ill and after she died, I tried to think of the good I could take from this experience. I know my mother wants me to go on and be strong and to grow from this. So I used it as an opportunity to grow. I really became a different person. I think that my reactions to things are different, my perceptions are differ-*

ent, my thinking and my priorities are different. The change has been extraordinary. It wasn't just because my mother died. That was the beginning of my change, or the beginning of a real desire for development and for growth. I had a real desire to learn, to understand, and to experience as much as I could.

Cynthia's most obvious move was ending a three-year relationship with her boyfriend. "I felt like it's one life, and you have to choose how you want your life to go. All of a sudden, I could see how fragile life really is. I saw my mom, and I saw how her life ended. She had lived much of her life feeling very bitter that she had gotten divorced, that she had been a single mother. She didn't think that was going to be her lot in life. I wanted to make the best of all my choices. I recognized that I was in the process of changing. I was beginning to look at who I was and what I wanted, and my boyfriend wasn't fitting in anymore."

Cynthia had always carried around pent-up anger, perhaps identifying with her mother's. But after her mother died, she actually became less angry inside.

I often look back at what I was like then and I think I've done a lot of work on myself. I used to be more insecure, defensive, and angry. Before my mother's illness, I was less conscious of others. Now I feel that connections are very important with my parents, brothers, my girlfriends, and my boyfriends; people are more important to me. I'm much more careful with people and more mindful of my friendships and my family. I try to be emotionally very healthy. I try to work out the issues that I have, rather than let them fester. I do a lot of yoga and meditation and try to lower my anxiety and fear, and do things that are nourishing to myself.

Many daughters try to make themselves or their lives different from those of their mothers' who had cancer, by improving their lifestyle habits or their attitude, as a way of warding off the impending threat of breast cancer, says psychologist and cancer survivor Roberta Hufnagel. Cynthia's mother chose not to face her cancer head on, but Cynthia says she would do it completely different if she were diagnosed. In fact, she has already begun to face cancer.

Recently, Cynthia began to volunteer at SHARE, a self-help support group in New York City for women with breast or ovarian cancer. Most of the women are patients themselves. Cynthia is one of only a few daughters. She works on the development committee, and once a month, she's an evening hostess, sitting behind the main desk and greeting women as they arrive for their support groups and as they leave to go home. "I've had some incredible experiences there. One woman came in, and she was about to take a cancer drug and wanted more information on it. I remembered seeing a video about the drug, and I took time to look for it. When I gave it to her, she said, 'You saved my life.' She hugged me and thanked me. I know I didn't save her life, but I felt like I had really helped somebody. If I can alleviate the pain of others and have my own suffering alleviated, that is great."

For Cynthia, the women at SHARE showed her a different way of dealing with cancer than her mother had. One evening, Cynthia was making copies for one of the volunteers, who had just had reconstructive surgery after having had a mastectomy. She said, "Do you want to see it?" and Cynthia said, "Sure," so she lifted up her shirt and said, "Doesn't this look great?" Cynthia agreed that it did. "In a lot of ways, it gave me hope if this should happen to me. These are women who are talking about it, they are strong and terrific and smart, and they don't look deformed or disfigured."

> *The last five years have been unbelievable. In a lot of ways, I'm really happy, because I think I turned what was a very difficult situation into something very beautiful, and even though my mom died, and I can't talk to her anymore, I feel like I have done the absolute best I can do with what happened, in terms of not hiding from it, not being bitter from it, and not having it overwhelm me. Instead, I'm out there trying to heal myself, to be there with other people, to be strong, and to remember my mom in ways*

that are significant. What is the point of this unless you can come out of it having grown, or having learned, or being available for someone else who is going through a similar situation? I don't feel sorry for myself. I feel really powerful in that I will be able to face anything that comes my way.

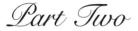

Part Two

TAKING CARE OF YOU

11

UNDERSTANDING
YOUR RISK

"My grandmother, aunt, and mother had breast cancer, which makes me completely vulnerable. I feel like it's just a question of when."

Suzanne Fiering, 36

*Y*ou have the same hair color as your mother, the same eyes, the same laugh, the same hips, but does that mean you will have the same medical fate? Many daughters of women with breast cancer think so. "I *know* that some day I'll get cancer," says Jennifer. "I *know* I'm going to lose my breasts," says Jill. "I feel like a walking time bomb," says Ellen. Daughters feel a powerful physical identification with their mothers, who are both genetically linked and gender linked. We feel such a strong physical connection that it is almost as if our bodies are a continuation of theirs. If we see mother has filled out in the hips, we think that our hips will follow in time; if we see certain distinctive wrinkles across her forehead, we think the same lines will emerge on our brows. So it would seem to follow, then, that daughters also feel they will get breast cancer, just like their mothers.

If you ask a daughter what her risk is, she'll almost always overestimate it. Three-fourths of women under age thirty who have a family history of breast cancer believe that they are likely to develop the disease someday, according to a study of high-risk women co-authored by Kathryn Kash of the Strang Cancer

Prevention Center. The study, published by the *Journal of the National Cancer Institute*, also found that among women of all ages with a first-degree relative (a mother, sister, or daughter) with cancer, 80 percent estimated their lifetime risk to be 50 percent or higher. In fact the average lifetime risk for this particular group of women was only 12 percent (about one in eight, which, by the way, is the average risk for women).

Overestimating your risk can be harmful in a variety of ways. It can play havoc on your state of mind and may even cause health problems. "It makes women more anxious and it makes them feel incredibly vulnerable and helpless about it," says Kash. These feelings, depending on how intense they are, can in turn affect how diligently you follow the recommendations for breast exams and mammography. Because some daughters fear that early detection tests will certainly find a tumor, they are more likely to avoid them altogether. Several studies have shown for some women that the greater your fear of breast cancer, the less likely you are to follow the guidelines for early detection—by either never going for your tests or skipping them for a couple of years. This may decrease the chances of detecting a cancer early and lower a woman's chance of survival if she does eventually discover a tumor.

The true risk for daughters is usually far below the perceived risk. In fact, the risk of a woman whose mother had breast cancer can actually be as low as one in eight—which is, as you probably know, the lifetime risk of the average American woman. How can a woman with a family history have a risk this low? The one-in-eight risk is an inclusive figure that already averages in very high-risk women with, say, a one in two risk, as well as very low-risk women with a one in fifteen risk. Therefore, you have to have a substantial number of risk factors for your odds to rise above average. Though having a mother with breast cancer is a risk factor, it may not dramatically increase your risk above the average, especially if you have no others. The misconception that anyone with a family history of cancer has a very high risk is perpetuated by the language used by the medical community and the media to describe these women. We mistakenly lump women with a family history together in a group called *high-risk women*.

Likewise, having a family history does not necessarily mean you have inherited one of the mutations of the BRCA1 (for BReast CAncer gene 1) and BRCA2 genes, the mutations that make women more susceptible to breast cancer and to ovarian cancer. You are likely to have a substantial family history (several members with breast cancer, a member who was diagnosed premenopausally, or a case of ovarian cancer) for there to be a chance that your mother's cancer is the hereditary type, rather than just random bad luck. Don't forget, cancer affects tens of thousands of women each year with no family history. Though estimates vary, only 6 to 19 percent of women who get breast cancer have a family history, says Jill Stopfer, MS, genetic counselor and familial cancer coordinator at the University of Pennsylvania. One case of cancer in your family, even if it's your mother's, simply does not mean your risk has jumped exponentially.

If you're someone who believes you're destined to get breast cancer, or even if you're not so fatalistic, going for risk counseling at a cancer center can be an important strategy for dealing with your emotions and your health. "If your risk turns out to be lower than you thought, it will make you feel a lot better. And if it's higher, which happens occasionally, you can start to develop a real surveillance program for yourself, and that can make you feel better as well," says UCLA psychologist David Wellisch. If you're right in your assessment, it can be a great relief to you to have a professional acknowledge that your fears are based on reality, that you're not being a hypochondriac, adds June Peters, the senior genetic counselor at the University of Pittsburgh.

Risk counseling typically consists of a *risk assessment,* which provides you with a percent risk and *counseling,* which addresses psychological issues that may be heightening your fear, as well as grief counseling, an early detection program, and prevention tactics you can take. Genetic risk counselors go through multidisciplinary training, including medical genetics, psychosocial theory, ethics, and counseling techniques. The counseling component should not be underestimated. If you simply layer risk statistics on top of your fears, it may do more damage than good, because you may interpret these figures through your own distorted lens. A study published in the *Journal of the National Cancer Institute* found that women with a family history who had high levels of anxiety about breast cancer risk did not improve their understanding of their risk after having simply a risk assessment. "As a counselor, I think it's a mistake to throw information about risk at people who have anxiety. It's better to talk about their feelings first, to validate that there are legitimate reasons they feel this way, and then examine some of the beliefs they have," says Peters. The harrowing memories about a mother's battle with cancer have to be verbalized and worked through before a person can step back and talk about her own risks, adds Peters. Women should leave risk counseling sessions with much more than a number. "Being given the opportunity to talk about being at risk can be very therapeutic," says Barbara Bernhardt, MS, genetic counselor of the Johns Hopkins Breast and Ovarian Surveillance Service.

For those reasons, genetic counselors are worried about the future of risk assessment. The mathematical models they use to calculate risk have become widely available to other health care workers, such as oncologists, OB/GYNs, and even internists and general practitioners, but these people won't be qualified to address the counseling issues. Likewise, genetic counselors are wary of the new "risk disk" available from the National Cancer Institute (NCI). Using this software, women can calculate their own risk. Experts worry that women who do their own risk assessments will also miss out on the counseling, and therefore may continue to hold onto their anxiety and may not fully comprehend their risk nor the early detection steps to take.

When you go for a risk assessment, the counselor will ask you about your family history, your personal medical history, and your lifestyle in order to pinpoint your risk factors. After running the numbers, she'll give you two figures, your lifetime risk and your risk for each decade of your life. Lifetime risk alone can be misleading, because women tend to assume that having, say, a 20 percent lifetime risk means they have a 20 percent risk of being diagnosed tomorrow, which is not at all the case because risk rises with age. Here's an example of how lifetime risk changes when it's calculated decade by decade. Say a twenty-nine-year-old woman is told she has a lifetime risk of 20 percent. When it's broken down by decade, her current risk at age twenty-nine is a fraction of a percent—0.7 percent. Her risk at age thirty-nine is 2 percent, her risk at forty-nine is 6 percent, her risk at fifty-nine is 10 percent (that's one in ten), her risk at sixty-nine is 16 percent, and finally, when and *if* she reaches eighty years old, that's when her risk will rise to 20 percent.

Counselors avoid offering relative risk figures, ratios that are bandied about routinely in the media. Relative risks are the numbers that show, for instance, that a woman who had her first period at age twelve has a 1.21 relative risk compared to someone who had her period at fourteen. Relative risks come from large epidemiological studies designed to find risk factors, but when women hear them, they mistakenly try to add their risk factors together, ending up with a frighteningly high and unrealistic figure. You can't add them together because the relative risk is specific to the study it came from, and complex mathematical equations are used to determine how these risk factors fit together.

Keep in mind that having risk factors, even several, does not necessarily mean you'll get the disease. It's a prediction, far from precise. "We have the ability to predict breast cancer only in a small group of people, those who have a hereditary risk where the risk is very high. But for the vast majority of people, we have no idea why one woman gets it and why someone doesn't," says Stopfer. Cancer is multifactorial, meaning that many environmental and genetic factors work together synergistically to either keep cancer from growing or promote it.

Though this chapter will not allow you to figure out your risk—that should only be done by a genetic risk counselor—it will explain the major risk factors that are typically considered during an assessment and give you a clear idea of which factors probably don't raise your risk very much and which probably do. With this information, you can take the appropriate steps to find your true risk and develop a screening program that is right for you, which is, after all, the reason risk counselors came to be in the first place. Other risks that have been less substantiated and haven't made it into these risk models will be discussed in Chapter 13, *Reducing Your Risk.*

THE RISKS

Gender and Age

Being female is your greatest risk factor. One in eight, or approximately 12.6 percent, of American women will develop breast
cancer during their lifetime. The second biggest risk factor is
aging. Despite frightening reports about young women developing breast cancer, the disease is highly uncommon in women in
their twenties and thirties. About 77 percent of breast cancers
occur in women over age fifty, according to the American Cancer
Society (ACS). But only 0.3 percent of breast cancer cases occur
in women in their twenties. A woman's chance of getting breast
cancer is about one in 2,525 by age thirty (see the chart below).

Risk of Breast Cancer by Age

Age	Risk
30	1 in 2,525
40	1 in 217
50	1 in 50
60	1 in 24
70	1 in 14
80	1 in 10
85	1 in 9
Over	1 in 8

Source: NCI Surveillance, Epidemiology, and End Results (SEER) Program.

Genetic Risk Factors

The third greatest risk is having a genetic mutation, which is not
like having cancer itself, but having a predisposition to cancer.
Recent studies have shown that about 10 percent or 18,000
breast cancer cases a year result from inherited mutations, or
changes in the BRCA1, BRCA2, or other as-yet-unidentified
genes. To provide some background on genetics, a gene is made
up of millions of the chemical bases, adenine (A), thymine (T),

cytosine (C), and guanine (G), which can be arranged in countless ways. These genes produce proteins that carry out specific functions in the cell. A gene has a mutation when one or more of the millions of bases has been knocked out of its correct place, or deleted, or added. Sometimes, long segments of bases are missing. Such an error throws off the genetic coding and can produce malfunctioning proteins. When functioning normally, the BRCA1 and BRCA2 genes, known as tumor suppressors, make proteins that inhibit malignant cells from multiplying. But if a person inherits a mutated gene from a parent, the mutation will produce damaged proteins that can't stem cancer growth but can give cancers the opportunity to gain a foothold.

It's estimated that one woman in 800 are born with a mutation in the BRCA1 or BRCA2 genes. BRCA mutations are more common in certain populations, like Ashkenazi Jewish women, who have a 1 in 40 chance of having a BRCA mutation, according to Stopfer. Women who inherit one of these mutations have a lifetime risk of developing breast cancer ranging from 35 percent to as high as 85 percent, as well as having a much greater risk of developing ovarian cancer. In the past, most women with a BRCA mutation were told their risk of breast cancer was between 65 and 85 percent. But these are now believed to be high estimates for the majority of mutation carriers. They were derived from the first hereditary cancer studies, which included families with many cases of breast cancer, whose members did have an exceedingly high risk. But for reasons not well understood, the incidence of cancer varies greatly among different populations and among different families with the mutation. One recent study of Ashkenazi Jewish women found that BRCA mutation carriers had a risk of 56 percent, and a new study from Iceland found that the risk among carriers was as low as 37 percent. Therefore, risk counselors need to take into consideration gene mutations as well as a woman's family history. The BRCA gene mutations are not the only ones that have been linked to breast cancer. Mutations of the p53, PTEN, and ATM genes are known to increase a woman's susceptibility to cancer, but they probably are responsible for a small number of cases. Testing for the mutations is an option more women are considering, though this is highly controversial. The pros and cons of testing are discussed in Chapter 12, *To Test or Not to Test.*

Family History

Perhaps the most widely known risk, and the most misunderstood, is having close relatives with breast cancer. While most women who have breast cancer in the family assume that this means they're doomed, risk can vary widely depending on the extent of their family history and the details of that history. Ideally, risk counselors delve into the last three generations, on both the mother's side of the family and the father's side. (Women often don't realize that the father's side imparts the same level of risk as the mother's.) A woman can still have a fairly low risk even if she has one or two close relatives with breast cancer. Risk doesn't begin to rise significantly until the number of relatives exceeds three or if someone in the family was diagnosed with cancer premenopausally or has ovarian cancer. These are the red flags that signal the cancer could be hereditary. Your risk also depends on the number of first-degree relatives vs. second-degree relatives (aunts, grandmothers, cousins), the type of breast cancer (there are many variations), the number of cancers found, and the history of ovarian cancer in your family.

In a study published in the *Journal of the American Medical Association* (JAMA), Stopfer and her coauthors divided women into two at-risk groups based on family history: moderate risk and high risk. Women who are at moderate risk have one to two close family members with breast cancer who were diagnosed postmenopausally and had no cases of ovarian cancer in the family. This group has a lifetime risk ranging from 12 to 30 percent. High-risk women in her study had at least three close relatives with breast cancer often diagnosed at an early age (younger than forty-five years), and possible ovarian cancer in the family. For high-risk women, their risk is 30 percent and higher. Take a look at the chart on page 147 to gain a better understanding of how your family history affects your lifetime risk.

This chart makes clear that the younger the women in your family were when diagnosed, the higher your risk; the more first-degree relatives with cancer in your family, the higher your risk; and the more women in your family who have cancer, the higher your risk. Also important, and somewhat encouraging, if the women in your family were diagnosed in their sixties and seventies (the majority of diagnoses), your risk barely rises above the average. Also, remember that your risk, like everyone else's, is much lower in the younger decades of your life. The chart on page 148 shows what your risk would be at age forty-nine depending on your family history.

A woman's predicted cumulative risk of breast cancer by age seventy-nine is based on the number of relatives and their age at diagnosis of cancer. Note: The risk at age seventy-nine for the general population is 10 percent.

Age of onset of relative's cancer	One second-degree relative	One first-degree relative	One first- and one second-degree relative	Two first-degree relatives with same age of onset
20–29	14.2	21.1	45.0	48.4
30–39	12.0	16.5	41.4	43.7
40–49	10.4	13.2	33.8	35.4
0–59	9.4	11.0	23.3	24.5
60-69	9.4	9.6	14.8	15.6
70-79	8.3	8.8	10.5	10.9

Note: These risks are derived from the popular risk prediction model called the Claus model. Figures may, however, underestimate the risk in mutation carriers and overestimate it in noncarriers. The chart is useful in providing an understanding of the risk increases based on the number of relatives and their ages at diagnosis.

A woman's predicted cumulative risk of breast cancer by age forty-nine is based on the number of relatives and their age at diagnosis of cancer. Note: The risk for the general population is 2 percent.

Age of onset of relative's cancer	One second-degree relative	One first-degree relative	One first- and one second-degree relative	Two first-degree relatives with same age of onset
20–29	3.5	6.2	15.3	16.6
30–39	2.7	4.4	13.9	14.8
40–49	2.1	3.2	11.0	11.7
50–59	1.7	2.3	7.0	7.5
60–69	1.7	1.8	3.8	4.1
70–79	1.3	1.5	2.1	2.3

Note: These risks are derived from the popular risk prediction model called the Claus model. Figures may, however, underestimate the risk in mutation carriers and overestimate it in noncarriers.

Breast History

Previous suspicious findings, whether from a mamogram or a biopsy, may affect a woman's risk of cancer. With the increased use of mammography, there has been a rise in the diagnosis of two breast abnormalities, ductal carcinoma in situ (DCIS) and lobular carcinoma in situ (LCIS). These abnormalities arise within the breast's lobules and ducts that make and transport milk. They usually pad the lining of the lobules and ducts but don't turn into palpable lumps themselves, so they're nearly impossible to detect by physical breast exams. Studies have found that LCIS rarely develops into cancer, though it can be a sign of an increased chance of breast cancer. A small percentage of DCIS do grow into cancers, but they are typically very slow-growing. Both abnormalities, however, are considered to be markers for cancer and they are associated with an increased risk of developing invasive breast cancer later in life. LCIS has a relative risk of 7.2, and DCIS, a relative risk of 11. In addition, a lump biopsy may raise your risk, though how much it rises depends on the results of the test. If the biopsy show atypical hyperplasia, meaning that there are low to moderately abnormal cells growing at an accelerated rate, a woman has a relative risk of 4.4. If the biopsy shows hyperplasia without atypia, meaning there is excess growth of cells with no sign of abnormal cells, she may have only a slightly higher risk of breast cancer. Lumpy breasts, in the past, erroneously referred to as fibrocystic breast disease, does not increase a woman's risk of cancer unless biopsies show that there are abnormal cells growing in those lumps, which is uncommon. Eighty percent of lumps that are biopsied in premenopausal women are benign.

X rays

Women who have had radiation therapy to the chest area earlier in their lives as treatment for Hodgkin's disease, non-Hodgkin's lymphoma, or any other reason are at an increased risk for breast cancer. Diagnostic X rays such as mammography are not believed to increase risk.

Reproductive Factors

A woman's lifelong exposure to estrogen has been linked to her risk. A woman's greatest exposure to estrogen comes with the steady ebb and flow of hormones that regulate her menstrual cycle. Women who started menstruating at an early age (before age twelve), thereby having had more cumulative exposure to estrogen, have a slightly elevated risk (a relative risk of 1.21 compared to those who began menstruating at age fourteen). Likewise, women who go through menopause at a late age (after age fifty-five) have a relative risk of 2.0.

Women who have had no children or who had their first child after age thirty have a higher breast cancer risk (a relative risk of 1.9 and 2.8, respectively), though the reasons for this association are not clear. Some theories suggest that until pregnancy, a woman's breasts are considered to be developing, and a developing breast may be more sensitive to carcinogens than a breast that has matured through pregnancy. Another theory is that the hormones of a pregnancy mature the healthy breast tissue in a young woman, but the same hormones of pregnancy in a woman older than thirty may actually stimulate malignancies that have already occurred in breast tissue, thus promoting cancer growth.

Other Risk Factors

Other factors, mostly linked to lifestyle, are thought to influence risk but are not taken into account in the models that calculate risk. Although important, they do not have a strong enough influence to be considered in these predictions. These risk factors will be discussed in Chapter 13, *Reducing Your Risk*.

12

TO TEST OR NOT
TO TEST

"I don't want to know; I don't need to know."

Jane Kistler, 39

*W*hen a test for a genetic mutation linked to breast cancer and ovarian cancer became available in 1994, it was hailed as one of the great advancements in cancer science, with the promise of identifying and saving the lives of those who harbor the gene mutations. This advancement, though, was a double-edged sword. Prior to genetic testing, the medically proactive among us subscribed to the adage "Knowledge is power." The more you knew about the details of your medical illnesses and treatments, the better off you would be, both psychologically and physically. But genetic testing gives us the ability to predict (to some degree) our medical fate, and the implications of that prediction are so complex, so controversial, and so potentially life-altering that now the medical pundits are saying *too* much knowledge may do you harm.

Indeed, the American Cancer Society (ACS) and the American Society of Human Genetics, along with many other major health organizations, strongly advise women to thoroughly understand and carefully weigh the benefits and risks of genetic testing before doing it. They have issued forceful statements to help counter the sometimes aggressive advertising of university cancer centers and genetic testing companies. The leading genetic experts worry that although we have the technology to test for genetic mutations, the medical community is lacking in its ability to provide adequate counseling to individuals. They don't know what to tell women about their medical choices; they don't have clear ethical guidelines; and they can't legally protect people who get tested.

Most of these medical associations agree that genetic testing for BRCA mutations is an option that should be reserved for only those women with a substantial family history—having several relatives with breast cancer or relatives who were diagnosed with breast cancer premenopausally, or those with ovarian cancer—in which case, there is a chance, albeit small, that they will test positive. For all other women, the chance of inheriting a mutation is so minute that it's not worth the emotional and financial cost. Women who qualify can't proceed with a test without first signing an informed consent form, a cautious step that is usually reserved for surgeries or experimental studies. Informed consent ensures that patients have been told about and fully understand all the benefits and risks of a procedure. "My concern is for people to get adequate counseling so that they come to an informed choice, whatever the choice may be," says Gladys Rosenthal, MS, genetic counselor at the Strang Cancer Prevention Center in New York City. Because of the drawbacks, many women are choosing not to get tested. Studies show that when high-risk women are given the option, about half want it and half don't. Those who are more likely to get tested are women with more extensive family histories, women who have anxiety about cancer, and those who are young.

Women seek genetic testing for a number of reasons. Some can't live with the uncertainty; to know their status gives them a sense of control over their life. Some hope to ease their anxiety by finding negative results or by looking for reassurance that their risks are not much higher than the average woman's. Some hope that if they test negative, they can avoid the expensive and emotionally taxing surveillance programs followed by high-risk women—regular breast exams, mammography, and ovarian cancer screening. On the other hand, if they test positive, they know they need to follow the program religiously. Some want to get tested for their children's sake. If a parent knows she's not a carrier, she can feel some relief that she has not passed on the mutations to her children. Some are looking for a biological explanation for their family's "bad luck" with cancer. For women who are contemplating prophylactic mastectomy or prophylactic oophorectomy (removal of the ovaries), the results of a test can help sway her one way or the other.

These are the benefits of gene testing. But the risks are just as weighty, and they're often not well understood by women who seek testing. "Most people we found who are interested in undergoing genetic testing have a limited knowledge of the disadvantages of the tests," says Robert T. Croyle, PhD, associate director for behavioral research with the Division of Cancer Control and Population Sciences at the National Cancer Institute. There is, for instance, the little known drawback that the test will be uninformative. Genetic testing is a complex, demanding process, and because it's in its infancy, many quirks and imperfections have not yet been worked out. If you recall from the last chapter, a mutation occurs when one or more bases—adenine, thymine, cytosine, and guanine, which form the gene's amino acids—have been deleted or inserted in the wrong place. To date, there are at least 500 known mutations on the BRCA1 and BRCA2 genes, but it's still a work in progress. The tests are not 100 percent accurate in picking up all alterations in these genes. They do miss insertions or deletions of genetic material, which would give a woman a false negative test result.

Another reason for a false negative result is that other gene mutations that have been linked to breast cancer, such as p53, PTEN, and ATM genes, are not yet being tested for (a test for p53 mutation exists, but it's not standard practice to test for this in high-risk women because it's rare). "The p53 and PTEN genetic mutations may be rare in breast cancer, but we think ATM is more common, and that there are others like it that have yet to be discovered," says June Peters, senior genetic counselor at the University of Pittsburgh. There may be a BRCA3. The only way to get a negative result that is conclusive is to belong to a family in which a mutation has been identified in others who have tested positive for it. You could request a test for that particular mutation, and if you test negative, then you know you don't have the mutation that has plagued your family.

Experts worry that women who get negative test results may feel a false sense of security and think they have no chance of getting cancer, even though they still have at least the same risk as the general population and still need to follow screening recommendations. Women with a strong family history who get an inconclusive negative result have to continue the stepped-up surveillance that's recommended for high-risk women. There's also the risk of getting neither a positive nor a negative result, which is not uncommon. This happens when the test detects a mutation, but it is not known whether that particular mutation affects the gene's functioning and increases your risk. "This can be a very upsetting result.... The women know they have something wrong, but they don't know if it will harm them," says Rosenthal.

A more widely known risk of genetic testing has to do with privacy and discrimination. If you test positive for a mutation, with the results in your medical records, there's no guarantee of privacy, and there is a chance that you could be discriminated against in several areas of your life. Health insurance companies could equate your gene mutation carrier status with having a pre-existing disorder and deny health insurance or charge you much higher rates. Providers of disability and life insurance may also be able to obtain your medical records and deny coverage. Or you may face discrimination in the workplace, by being either turned down for a job or fired, because of an employer's fear that providing you with health insurance may cost a bundle. Some women deal with this issue by making their doctors swear that they won't enter their genetic status into their medical records. Some are so worried about discrimination that they give their genetic counselors fake names and pay for the test with a money order, so there's no way to trace their name.

In the future, women who carry mutations won't have to cover their tracks as if they were fugitives. Federal and state legislators are working to pass laws to prevent this kind of discrimination and invasion of privacy. The federal Health Insurance

Portability and Accountability Act of 1996 offers some protection for those in group health insurance plans, but consumer advocates believe it's inadequate, and legislators are working on more comprehensive bills. At the state level, as of August 1998, twenty-eight states have laws restricting health insurance discrimination, so be sure to ask about these laws in your state. The Americans with Disabilities Act and the Equal Employment Opportunity Commission may protect carriers of mutations from discrimination, but these laws have not yet been tested in the courts.

Aside from the legal risks, a more immediate risk is to your emotional health. Researchers are actively studying the psychological consequences of genetic testing. Studies show that simply deciding to test can result in high levels of anxiety, depression, sleep difficulties, and other problems, says Peters. If a woman tests negative, that can ease a lot of her anxieties, though it can take a long time for the news to sink in. "Some women can't believe they're negative because for so long, they have assumed that they're at very high risk, just waiting for the other shoe to drop," says genetic counselor Gladys Rosenthal of the Strang Cancer Prevention Center. If a woman tests positive, however, she may find it much harder to cope. In a study of depression in high-risk women, conducted by Caryn Lerman from the Lombard Cancer Center at Georgetown University Medical Center in Washington, D.C., the rate of depression for those who tested negative was 8 percent, compared with 14 percent in those who tested positive. "When you're telling a woman she has the gene mutation, it appears to have the same sort of psychological impact as telling a woman she has cancer," says Barbara Bernhardt, genetic counselor for the Johns Hopkins Breast and Ovarian Surveillance Service. "It's a crisis, but women do over time incorporate that information into their lifestyle and get on with their lives," she adds. Even when some women test positive, they actually feel a sense of relief because knowing is far better than living with uncertainty. Uncertainty tends to make us feel that things are out of our control.

In fact, Lerman's research found that for some women, choosing *not* to get tested has worse consequences than getting a positive result. The women in Lerman's study who chose not to get tested had the highest rates of depression—19 percent compared with 14 percent of those who learned they were mutation carriers. The effects were worse for a sub-group of women who were very anxious about cancer prior to entering the study. In anxious women who turned down the test, depression rates jumped from 26 to 47 percent, whereas the depression rates stayed the same in anxious women who tested positive for the mutation—hovering around 20 percent. These results suggest that if you're extremely anxious about cancer, choosing not to get tested might increase your risk of depression, but if you have moderate anxiety, getting tested could make you depressed if you test positive.

Unfortunately, you're not the only person who will be affected by the results of your test. "The decision to get tested has repercussions for other family members, husbands, boyfriends, grown-up children, sisters, and even cousins," says Rosenthal. A mantra among genetic counselors is "The patient is the *family*." Says Croyle, "People need to be aware of the fact that genetic information is unique in that it says something not only about the person being tested but also about her blood relatives." A relative might not want to know her genetic status but can learn about it involuntarily because another family member has gone through testing. These conflicts have caused rifts in families. It's not uncommon for different members of the same family to disagree on whether or not they should undergo testing. Once they learn a family member carries a mutation, they may also disagree on whether they should reveal the results to other family members or to their physicians. Another issue that crops up in families is that some members may suffer from a phenomenon similar to survivor's guilt. They may actually feel guilty if they test negative when a sibling or a mother tests positive. Sometimes, different test results can cause an emotional divide between siblings because they no longer share the same life-threatening circumstances prior to the test.

The main questions you should ask yourself before getting tested are: What will you do with the results? What do you want to get out of testing? Would you do anything differently if you tested positive? Would you change the management of your health? Aside from early detection, which can increase the chances of surviving cancer, currently there is no proven way to prevent getting cancer. A few options may reduce risk, such as taking the drug tamoxifen or undergoing prophylactic mastectomy, but these are both fairly drastic measures with serious drawbacks and risks. (See discussion in Chapter 13, *Reducing Your Risk.*) If you know you won't opt for either, it may not be worth getting tested unless you know that finding out your genetic status will ease your anxiety or you're getting tested for the sake of another person in your family, like a daughter. Genetic counselors often advise women who are grieving their mother's death or are otherwise distraught to postpone the decision for several months until the intensity of their emotions fades.

The ACS recommends that if you're considering testing, first talk to a genetic counselor or other medical professional who's qualified to interpret and explain the implications of these tests. "A major concern that I have is that many primary care physicians can now request cancer genetic test through commercial routes, but they may have very limited knowledge about genetics and the psychological issues and medical issues related to a genetic test," says Croyle. Genetic counseling includes psychological support, guidance on early detection, and medical options, as well as referrals to doctors and surgeons. In the future, deciding to get tested may not be such an excruciating process. Steps are being taken to improve the reliability and accuracy of the tests, research is creating viable ways to cut your risk through drugs like tamoxifen, and legal measures are being taken to protect you from discrimination.

13

REDUCING YOUR RISK

"I try to dwell on the choices I have made in my life that are different from my mother's."

Cynthia Cohen, 31

Where there is breast cancer in mothers, there is fatalism in daughters. Where there is one diagnosis of cancer, daughters expect other diagnoses to follow. Many daughters fully believe that they will get the disease themselves. They believe there's nothing much they can do to alter their doomed course, as if they have been drawn into the powerful current of treacherous rapids. Certainly there isn't any vaccine or miraculous drug that women can take to prevent breast cancer, and because cancer is caused by a number of colliding events, scientists cannot pinpoint definitive strategies that will protect you. However, women can take certain steps that will definitely reduce their chances of dying from cancer, and there are things they can do that may reduce their chances of getting cancer in the first place. In fact, at the same time that daughters are feeling the pull of a morbid fate, many are furiously backpedaling against it by making changes that are in their control—following early diagnosis guidelines, watching their diet, not drinking alcohol, and avoiding synthetic estrogens. Aside from the health benefits they get from taking these steps, daughters feel better emotionally regaining a sense of control over a disease that tends to leave people feeling otherwise helpless.

But not all daughters take control. There is great concern among experts in this field that women with a family history are too afraid to follow important guidelines, especially early detection tests. Based on her studies of high-risk women, the Strang Center's Kathryn Kash says, "The more anxious women were about cancer, the less often they came in for mammography and clinical breast exams." Her studies found a direct correlation between fear and screening behaviors. "The less fear they had, the more they did. The more fear, the less they did," says Kash. It's human nature to avoid what we fear, and some daughters are so certain that these tests might actually find a lump that they avoid them altogether. But there's hope for even overly anxious daughters. Kash did a pilot study in which high-risk women attended six group sessions that provided information about breast cancer from oncologists and risk counselors, and support from other women in the group. "We found that women who came to the sessions felt well connected to each other, well connected to the breast cancer center, less anxious about getting breast cancer, better able to cope, and were more likely to do breast self-exam and follow other screening guidelines," says Kash. She hypothesizes that if women educate themselves about their risk of breast cancer and if they talk to others about their fears, they are less likely to be afraid and more likely to catch a tumor in its early stages. "You have to be proactive about your health, not sit back and say 'I don't want to think about breast cancer,'" says Kash.

Regular Mammograms

It squashes your breasts, it's embarrassing, and it may fill you with dread, but mammography is the leading component of early detection. As many daughters know from their experiences with their mother's cancer, the earlier you detect a tumor, the better your chances of survival. The goal is to find cancers early, before they have had the opportunity to metastasize, or spread, to other organs and other areas of the body, where they can threaten your life.

A routine mammogram consists of two X rays of each breast. The images can detect tumors five millimeters in size and sometimes find tumors as small as one millimeter. Several clinical trials have found that regular mammography can decrease the chance of dying from breast cancer in women ages fifty to sixty-nine by about one third. Aside from the lifesaving benefits of mammography, a woman who finds a tumor early may be able to choose breast-conserving surgery, a lumpectomy, rather than undergo a mastectomy, which removes the entire breast. Moreover, a woman may only have to undergo lumpectomy and radiation therapy, thereby avoiding chemotherapy.

Whether or not younger women, under fifty years old, reap benefits from mammography has been a hotly debated question, one for which there is no consensus among the country's leading cancer authorities. There certainly is a need for early detection in younger women, as about 23 percent of all breast cancers occur in women under age fifty. That equals about 41,600 younger women each year who are diagnosed—no small statistic. Mammography has its benefits over physical breast exams. Some studies have found that tumors detected by mammographic screening of women in their forties were smaller and at an earlier stage, in other words, more treatable, than cancers found in women of the same age who weren't having mammography. Theoretically, since tumors found in younger women tend to be more aggressive, catching them early can make a life-and-death difference.

Mammography, however, is not always reliable in young women and may come with risks. A mammogram detects tumors by highlighting dense clusters of cells, which show up white on the image. But the breast tissue in younger women, which is very dense, also appears white on the X ray, so it can obscure a cancer. Mammograms miss up to 25 percent of all breast cancers in women under fifty, compared with missing 10 percent of cancers in women in their fifties. When a mammogram doesn't detect a cancer, the report is called a false negative, a result that can have serious consequences. There's concern among experts that young women who get negative mammograms are lulled into a false sense of safety and will ignore lumps they may find on their own, dismissing them as benign without getting an expert opinion. Experts also worry about false positive results—when abnormalities detected on mammograms turn out to be benign in follow-up biopsy testing. For every eight biopsies performed in women in their forties, one invasive breast cancer and one *in situ* cancer (a less serious tumor contained within a milk-producing lobule or duct) is found, according to the National Institutes of Health's *Consensus Statement: Breast Cancer Screening for Women Ages 40–49.* But during the days and sometimes weeks of follow-up testing, those six out of eight women who had the false positives had to go through emotional hell, fearing they had cancer, fearing they would lose their breasts, and fearing they might die.

Whether mammography actually reduces the number of deaths from breast cancer in younger women is not definitely known. In support of mammography, the *Journal of the National Cancer Institute* published a meta-analysis of five large-scale studies in 1997, which found a 29 percent reduction in mortality for women ages forty to forty-nine who got regular mammograms. Some studies, however, show a greater reduction while others show no reduction at all. These inconsistencies, which may be blamed on flaws in the study designs, make it difficult for the leading cancer organizations to agree on mammography for younger women.

The American Cancer Society (ACS) recommends that all women over forty have a mammogram once a year. The National Cancer Institute (NCI) recommends that women between the ages of forty and forty-nine get mammograms every one to two years and that women fifty years old and over have one done annually. However, both the ACS and the NCI advise women with a family history of breast cancer to consult their doctors about earlier and more frequent tests.

The country's leading cancer experts published a consensus statement in the *Journal of the American Medical Association* (JAMA) offering recommendations for women who have inherited a mutation in the BRCA1 or BRCA2 gene, or for those who are suspected of having a mutation because others in their family have tested positive. They recommend annual mammography beginning somewhere between the ages of twenty-five to thirty-five. The decision of when to get your first mammogram should be made by you and your doctors, based on various factors such as awareness of the limitations of mammography in younger women, effectiveness of physical exams on your breasts by you and your doctor, and the risks of mammography, such as false negative and false positive results. The JAMA statement goes on to warn that there is a potential, though not a proven, increased risk of breast cancer in women who begin mammography at an early age, because their breasts may be more sensitive to radiation. Women who have the gene mutation may be even more susceptible to the effects of radiation, although they are the ones who need early detection the most. The amount of radiation in a mammogram is less than one rad, comparable to what you'd be exposed to if you took a flight from New York to California. Most experts believe the benefits of early mammography outweigh the risks, and most physicians and genetic risk counselors at cancer prevention centers base their advice for mutation carriers on the JAMA consensus statement.

Breast Exams

Because mammography cannot find all breast cancers, the ACS and the NCI also recommend physical breast exams—that is, palpating the breast for suspicious lumps with the fingertips—conducted by your gynecologist or breast specialist. Ten percent of breast cancers are detected by health care providers, so physical examination is still considered an important part of your early detection program. It's particularly important in younger women, for whom mammography is less reliable because of their dense breasts. The ACS recommends that women ages twenty to forty have a physical breast exam every three years and all women forty years old and over have a physical breast exam once a year. For women with a family history and those with a BRCA1 or BRCA2 gene mutation, annual or semiannual breast exams are recommended beginning at age twenty-five to thirty-five years old.

You know the feel of your breasts better than anyone, and the more regularly you do breast self-examination (BSE), the more likely you'll notice a change in them. Studies show that many breast irregularities or abnormalities are found by women themselves, though the majority of these irregularities are benign.

Although there is no conclusive evidence that BSE saves lives, there are many anecdotal reports of women who say they found their cancer themselves through BSE, in some cases only months after having a "clean" mammogram. Monthly BSE is recommended for all women, beginning early in life (age eighteen to twenty-one), to help establish regular habits and familiarize women with the feel and appearance of their own breasts.

Try to perform BSE at the same time every month. The best time is right after your period, because breasts are usually the least tender and least lumpy (benign cysts tend to enlarge before your period, making it difficult to know what's normal and what's not). If you do not have regular periods or sometimes skip a month, do BSE on the same day every month. It's a good idea to ask your physician to demonstrate the correct method of BSE. The ACS recommends the following steps.

1. Lie down with a pillow under your right shoulder and place your right arm behind your head.
2. Use the pads on the three middle fingers on your left hand to feel for lumps in the right breast.
3. Press firmly enough to know how your breast feels. A firm ridge in the lower curve of each breast is normal.
4. Move around the breast in a circular, up-and-down line, or wedge pattern. Be sure to do it the same way every time, check the entire breast area, and remember how your breast feels from month to month.
5. Repeat the exam on your left breast (move the pillow under your left shoulder).
6. Repeat the exam of both breasts while standing, with one arm behind your head. The upright position makes it easier to check the upper and outer part of the breasts (toward your armpit, which is where about half of breast cancers are found). You may want to do the exam in the shower— soapy water makes it easier to do.
7. Stand in front of a mirror and check your breast for any dimpling of the skin, changes in the nipple, redness, or swelling.

Be sure to call your gynecologist or a breast specialist if you notice any changes in your breasts. While the vast majority of lumps are benign, they all should be checked by a physician.

Reprinted with pemission of the American Cancer Society, Inc.

Exposure to Estrogens

One of the most widely studied risk factors for breast cancer is a woman's lifelong exposure to the female hormone estrogen. As discussed in earlier chapters, factors such as the age a woman begins menstruating and the age she enters menopause—two events that turn on and off the flow of estrogen—affect her over-all risk. Many types of breast cancers are stimulated by estrogen, so the more the cells of your body are exposed to the hormone, the greater the chance that aberrant cells will grow. Because of this proven relationship, much attention has also been paid to a woman's exposure to exogenous estrogens such as oral contraceptives and hormone replacement therapy (HRT) taken for menopause. Despite the intense scrutiny of these hormone medications, experts cannot say with certainty that they greatly increase risk.

Oral Contraceptives

Numerous studies examining oral contraceptives as a risk factor for breast cancer have produced—for the most part—inconsistent results. Some studies have found that taking birth control pills, which contain estrogen and progestin, does raise breast cancer risk, although the increase is small and appears to have a short-term effect. A meta-analysis of data from fifty-four studies worldwide, involving about 53,300 women with breast cancer and 100,240 women without breast cancer identified a slightly elevated risk (relative risk of 1.24) of developing breast cancer for current users of birth control pills and an even smaller risk for those who had stopped using the pills one to four years earlier (relative risk of 1.16). The meta-analysis, which was published in the prestigious journal *The Lancet*, found that the inceased risk disappeared with time. About ten years after stopping use of oral contraceptives, no increased risk was seen. This return to normal after ten years occurred in all women, including those with a family history of breast cancer and regardless of the type of birth control pill taken, the dose, or the length of time on the pill.

Other studies have found that long-term use of oral contraceptives leads to a greater risk. A study in the *Journal of the National Cancer Institute* found that women who used birth control pills for ten years or more had a higher relative risk (1.3) than those who never used them. Likewise, women who started birth control pills early in life—within five years of their first period—had the same elevated risk (1.3).

On the other hand, there are benefits associated with birth control pills, aside from their obvious and intended use for contraception. Several studies have shown a reduced risk—as much as 60 percent—of ovarian cancer in women who took oral contraceptives, which is an important benefit for women who have inherited a BRCA gene mutation, a significantly increased risk for ovarian cancer.

There is still not enough solid information to make a blanket recommendation for women or to issue a warning. A 1995 study conducted by Kent Hoskins, MD, and fellow researchers at the University of Pennsylvania and the Dana Farber Cancer Institute in Boston recommended that all women at increased risk of breast cancer avoid use of exogenous estrogens when possible. Though the authors state that this recommendation may prove overzealous in the future, they write, "in the absence of data, we have chosen to abide by the Hippocratic principle of 'First, do no harm.'" For those with a proven genetic mutation, it's an even tougher choice. "It's a difficult decision because the Pill does decrease the risk for ovarian cancer, and many of these women who are at risk for breast cancer are also at risk for ovarian cancer," says Sue Miesfeldt, MD, the director of the Cancer Genetics Clinic at the University of Virginia Health Sciences Center. "If you really don't need to use estrogen, I wouldn't recommend it," she adds.

Most experts agree that more studies are needed to fully understand the relationship between oral contraceptives and breast cancer, especially since the amount of estrogen used in oral contraceptives has been reduced in the past few decades. However, because the research does show a slight increased risk, you should discuss use of oral contraceptives with your physician and determine whether it's a slight risk worth taking.

Hormone Replacement Therapy

The risks of taking hormone therapy are more established than those for oral contraceptives. Some women may choose to take estoogen or a combination of estrogen and progestin to relieve the symptoms of menopause, which can include hot flashes, sleep disturbances, and vaginal discomfort (only about 25 percent of women who reach menopause get these annoying symptoms, studies show). HRT has also been recommended to women because it may reduce loss of bone density associated with osteoporosis. Some studies have shown that it may decrease the risk of cardiovascular disease, though this finding has not been proven in a controlled clinical trial.

Duing the last twenty-five years, more than fifty epidemiological studies have examined the effect HRT may have on the incidence of breast cancer, but the results are mixed. Studying HRT is difficult on many fronts. Many of the older studies have followed women who used high doses of estrogen alone, while today many women take a combination of estrogen and progestin, which may or may not increase risk more. Demographically, women who choose to take HRT tend to have a lower risk of breast cancer to begin with—for instance, they tend to be on the thin side, which lowers risk. This bias in the study population would lead to a lower incidence of breast cancer in the studies compared with the general population, and therefore a low estimate of the effects of HRT.

Several studies have found that women who take HRT for fewer than five years do not appear to have an increased risk. There is, however, increasing evidence that women who take HRT over the long term do see a rise in their risk. In a meta-analysis of fifty-one studies and 150,000 women that was published in *The Lancet*, researchers found that for each year a woman is on HRT, her risk of breast cancer increases by 2.3 percent. (These studies were done on women who took estrogen without progestin.) For those who had taken estrogen for five years or longer (the average being eleven years), they had a thirty-five times greater risk of breast cancer than the general population. However, the risks may not apply to past users of HRT. One recent study found that a woman's breast cancer risk returns to that of the general population within five years of stopping.

Some physicians and researchers believe that the benefits of HRT—alleviating menopause systems and lowering the risk of osteoporosis and possibly heart disease—outweigh the risks associated with breast cancer. "You don't want to deny a woman the benefit associated with hormone replacement therapy if there's little evidence that it's harmful," says Gladys Rosenthal, genetic counselor with the Strang Center in New York City. At the same time, Rosenthal adds, many physicians do not prescribe HRT for women with a family history of breast cancer. They want more definitive proof that HRT isn't a risk.

They are waiting for a double-blind, placebo-controlled clinical trial, the gold standard of scientific research, in which one group is given HRT and one group placebo, and both groups are followed for many years. A study of this type, called the Women's Health Initiative, is underway but won't conclude for several years. Until then, whether a woman should take HRT and, if so, for how long should be the individual's decision, based on her family history, her risks of breast cancer, her risks of heart disease and osteoporosis, and other lifestyle factors. Some women who decide against HRT may prefer to take other steps to reduce their risks of osteoporosis and heart disease, including exercising, losing weight, healthy eating, and taking vitamin E, folate, and calcium supplements.

Your Weight

If you're postmenopausal, one impotant step to take is to bring your weight down to the normal range. Being overweight is a proven risk factor for breast cancer in postmenopausal women. Fat cells are thought to metabolize androgens (male hormones) into estrogens in older women, thus raising levels of estrogen in the body, which promotes tumor growth. The risk seems to be higher for overweight women who have never taken hormone replacement therapy (the rise in estrogen levels by being over-weight is obscured by the increase caused by HRT). Being over-weight also increases the risk of not surviving breast cancer if you're diagnosed, in both premenopausal and postmenopausal women.

Whether or not younger, premenopausal women also bene-fit from losing weight is not known. There isn't compelling evi-dence that premenopausal women who are overweight are at a greater risk of getting breast cancer than others, and in fact, being heavy when you're younger has been shown to be slightly protective. Experts theorize that overweight women are more likely to experience anovulation, that is, skipping periods, which lowers their lifetime exposure to estrogen. The same is true of women who are underweight.

What may be more important than your current weight is your weight gained since you were eighteen years old. The Harvard Nurses' Health Study of more than 95,000 women ages thirty to fifty-five, who were followed for sixteen years, found that women who gained forty-four pounds or more after age eighteen had a 40 percent higher risk of developing breast cancer after menopause than women who gained only four or five pounds. The study also concluded that weight gain of more than five pounds since the age of eighteen accounted for approximate-ly 16 percent of all breast cancers in postmenopausal women.

Exercise

Exercise is a key component to any weight loss and weight maintenance program, which is an important goal for postmeno-pausal women. But vigorous exercise may also have an effect on breast cancer risk. Exercise may lower the levels of estrogen cir-culating in your body, thus lowering risk. One study published in the *New England Journal of Medicine* examined the work and leisure activities of about 25,600 pre- and post-menopausal women. It found that women who exercised at least four hours a week had a 37 percent reduction in the risk of breast cancer. Among premenopausal women, their risk dropped 47 percent.

Nonetheless, there's no consensus on exercise either. An analysis of the exercise habits of more than 100,000 women participating in the Harvard Nurses' Health Study, which is one of the most telling studies we have, found no reduction in risk in women who exercised more during high school or who currently exercised more. Critics of the study claim it looked at only two limited time periods and did not measure lifelong fitness practices. What is indisputable, however, is that adolescents who exercise have a lower risk of breast cancer. Researchers believe that the physical activity can delay menarche (a girl's first period) and interrupt the menstrual cycle, thus lowering a woman's lifetime exposure to estrogen. That's a convincing argument for encouraging young daughters of women with breast cancer to get out on the playing field.

Obtaining health benefits from exercise does not require a tremendous amount of effort. The general guideline of the American College for Sports Medicine, the authorities on exercise, is to work out four or five times a week for about thirty minutes. Ideally, you should incorporate three different types of exercise into your weekly schedule: aerobic exercising, strength-building, and flexibility (stretching or yoga). The health benefits of exercise can be achieved by women of any age, so it is never too late to start.

Low-Fat, High-Fiber Diet

Breast cancer risk has also been linked to the fat in your diet, but again, the studies are often contradictory. They don't necessarily explain what types of fat are bad or whether it's simply the excess calories we get from fat, or the components of the fat itself that is the problem. Although there's no good explanation for how fat in food promotes cancer, most experts agree that a high-fat diet can increase the risk. Their opinion is supported by comparisons of the incidence of cancer and the amount of dietary fat in the diets of different countries. Breast cancer is typically lower in countries with low-fat diets, and data show that as these countries, such as Japan, eat a more Westernized diet—a higher fat diet—the rate of breast cancer increases. Of course, these studies are not definitive because the rise could be explained by other population-wide factors, such as Japan's more Westernized lifestyle—more stress and more pollution.

The fat connection may actually be a fiber connection. Diets that are high in fat tend to be low in fiber, and fiber is believed to be important in lowering cancer risks. Studies have also found that high-fiber diets are linked to lower estrogen levels circulating in the body, which protect against breast cancer.

Experts recommend lowering fat intake to less than 20 percent of your calories (studies in rats found that as the rats' fat intake rose above 20 percent, their rates of breast cancer began to rise). To maintain a low-fat diet, try to choose lean cuts of meat, skinless poultry, or fresh fish; select nonfat or low-fat milk, yogurt, and cheese. Ask for low-fat salad dressings; use low-fat cooking methods such as baking or roasting rather than frying and sautéing. When you need to use fat for cooking, make it a monounsaturated oil such as olive oil or canola oil, recommends Marguerite Eng, an oncology nutritionist for the Don Monti Cancer Center at the North Shore Hospital in Manhasset, New York. Avoid hydrogenated oils and vegetable oils such as corn oil, soybean oil, and safflower-seed oil.

Increase the amount of fiber-rich fruits and vegetables you eat, aiming for at least five servings a day. These foods are also loaded with cancer-protective antioxidants. Eng recommends eating fruits and vegetables high in beta-carotene and alpha-carotene, such as carrots, sweet potatoes, spinach, kale, and cantaloupe, as well as cruciferous vegetables such as broccoli and cauliflower. Sample servings include one-half cup of raw vegetables, a piece of medium-sized fruit, or one-quarter cup of dried fruit.

Drinking and Smoking

Alcohol is linked to an increased risk of developing breast cancer. Compared with nondrinkers, women who consume one alcoholic drink a day have a small increase in risk, and those who have two to five drinks daily, regardless of the type of drink, have 1.4 times the risk of women who drink no alcohol. The effect of alcohol on breast cancer can also be traced to estrogen. It is believed to increase estrogen levels circulating in the body. The ACS recommends limiting your consumption of alcohol if you drink at all.

While no studies have yet linked cigarette smoking to breast cancer, smoking affects overall health and increases the risk for other cancers as well as heart disease. The toxic chemicals in cigarette smoke can also deplete levels of antioxidant nutrients, which defeats the purpose of eating more fruits and vegetables. Smoking can also limit the ways in which breast cancer can be treated.

Preventing Cancer with Drugs

In October 1998, the Food and Drug Administration (FDA) approved tamoxifen, brand name Nolvadex, for the reduction of the incidence of breast cancer in high-risk women. The approval was based on the results from the Breast Cancer Prevention Trial (BCPT), a nationwide study of 13,388 high-risk women. The study found that tamoxifen, an anti-estrogen, taken for about five years reduces the incidence of breast cancer by 44 percent in women aged thirty-five to forty-nine years, by 51 percent in women in their fifties, and by 55 percent in women aged sixty years and older.

Tamoxifen has been on the market since 1978 as a treatment for breast cancer. The drug fights cancer, primarily by attaching to the estrogen receptors on breast cancer cells. By taking up most of the cell's receptors, it essentially blocks out the body's estrogen that would normally have attached to these receptors and stimulated the malignant cells. These cells, then, don't get their estrogen boost, and over time their growth is inhibited, if not stalled altogether.

Despite its possible benefits, tamoxifen has serious side effects. According to the study, women taking the drug had more than twice the risk of developing endometrial cancer than those on the placebo, they had three times the risk of developing a life-threatening pulmonary embolism (a blood clot in the lung), and they were also more likely to have deep vein thrombosis (blood clots in major veins) as well as some less serious side effects including eye problems, depression, hot flashes, vaginal discharge, and bloating. Given the potentially life-threatening risks of taking tamoxifen, consumer advocates worry that the FDA approval was premature. Because the study was for only five years, they worry that the drug didn't actually prevent breast cancer but simply slowed the progression of existing tumors that were undetectable at the start of the study. Though that's certainly worthwhile, it may not be worth the risks and the expense— Nolvadex costs between $80 to $100 a month.

According to the FDA, only women with a particularly high risk qualify to take Nolvadex. A woman qualifies when her risk factors, after input into a mathematical model, show that her risk of developing breast cancer during a five-year is period at least 1.7 percent. This is the equivalent of the risk of a sixty-year-old woman without any other additional risk factors, meaning that most women in their sixties would qualify. The younger you are, the more risk factors you'll need to qualify. To provide some perspective, a forty-year-old woman would need the equivalent risk factors of one first-degree relative with breast cancer *plus* a history of two benign breast biopsies *plus* not having her first child until she was thirty years old or older *plus* getting her first period at the age of eleven or younger. That's a lot of risk factors.

In the future, tamoxifen won't be the one and only breast cancer prevention drug around. Pharmaceutical companies are racing to find other drugs, and one of the most promising is raloxifene, which is already approved for use in treating osteoporosis. Raloxifene may have a similar effect as tamoxifen, with fewer risks and side effects. An analysis of 7,705 women who participated in an osteoporosis treatment and fracture prevention study showed a 70 percent reduction in the incidence of newly diagnosed invasive breast tumors among the women who had taken raloxifene versus the placebo group. Similar to tamoxifen, the drug blocks the action of estrogen. But it is a selective estrogen receptor modulator (SERM), so it affects organs differently, having estrogenic effects on bone and lipid tissue, but anti-estrogenic effects on cells in the breast and the uterus. Therefore, unlike tamoxifen, raloxifene did not appear to increase the risk of endometrial cancer. A large-scale research project comparing the two drugs with each other, the Study of Tamoxifen and Raloxifene (STAR), which will include an estimated 22,000 postmenopausal women, is expected to begin in early 1999.

Prophylactic Mastectomy

Prophylactic mastectomy, or the removal of breasts in a woman who doesn't have cancer, is a highly controversial way of preventing breast cancer. Most women who are considering prophylactic mastectomy have tested positive for the genetic mutation or have several family members who have had breast cancer, and therefore have an extremely high risk of developing breast cancer themselves. Even among these women, however, the choice is still uncommon. According to one study, fewer than 6 percent of women who undergo gene testing would have the procedure done if they tested positive. Because of the negative psychological effects mastectomies can potentially cause the risks associated with surgery, the potential disfigurement that's involved, and the lack of a guarantee, any woman who chooses to remove her healthy breasts must have compelling reasons to do so.

Many women considering prophylactic mastectomy have witnessed their mothers battle breast cancer and eventually die from the disease. The experience was so horrifying for them that they often suffer from a debilitating fear of meeting the same fate. The fear is pervasive, affecting their day-to-day existence, their relationships, and many of their decisions. "Many worry that because their mother's breast cancer was diagnosed early, they thought they had beaten it, and then they died anyway. They think, no matter what I do, even if breast cancer is found early, I'll get it and die," says Barbara Bernhardt, genetic counselor of the Johns Hopkins Breast and Ovarian Surveillance Service. "They don't see early diagnosis as a viable route, they don't see breast cancer as something they will survive, so they see their only option is to remove their breasts." The procedure may also be recommended for high-risk women with breast calcifications (small calcium deposits that can be detected by mammography) or for high-risk women whose breast tissue is very dense. For those women, early detection of tumors by mammography may be extremely difficult.

Aside from reducing the fear in women undergoing breast removal, the surgery will also reduce their actual chance of dying from breast cancer. There's no guarantee, though, that it will prevent cancer from occurring. A 1997 consensus paper on follow-up recommendations for women who tested positive for the genetic mutation, published in JAMA, concluded that there isn't enough evidence to recommend for or against the procedure. A major reason for the authors' hesitancy in recommending it is that it's not foolproof. In a typical prophylactic mastectomy, the surgeon removes nearly all of the breast tissue, but a small amount always remains (less than five percent of breast tissue). There are thousands of breast cells on a pinpoint of tissue, and all it takes is one to turn malignant. Experts worry that breast cancer can develop in the remaining tissue. Based on four large studies, researchers found that high-risk women who undergo the surgery have a 1.18 percent chance of developing cancer, far below their risk if they hadn't had the procedure, but not perfect.

A 1999 study published in the *New England Journal of Medicine* found that the procedure reduced the risk of breast cancer in moderate to high risk women by about 90 percent. In the retrospective study led by Lynn Hartmann, MD, an oncologist at the Mayo Clinic in Rochester, Minnesota, the medical histories of 639 women who had had the procedure between 1960 and 1993 were analyzed. Of these women, seven developed breast cancer in the chest wall, and two eventually died from the disease. "The study is not to be a universal recommendation for prophylactic mastectomy to high risk women. It just provides data in a controversial area. The decision to proceed with this procedure is a complex and personal one," says Hartmann.

Aside from the lower risk, the procedure can improve a woman's quality of life by providing relief from the constant fear of cancer, from the continual examination of her breasts for lumps, and from the panic caused by anything the least bit unusual.

It is impossible to determine medically whether this surgery is the right choice for any particular woman. Some women with BRCA mutations may never develop breast cancer. A study published in the *New England Journal of Medicine* found that by age seventy, 44 percent of mutation carriers had not developed a breast cancer. These women would obviously not have benefited from the surgery. Other women who had prophylactic mastectomy learned after the surgery that their breasts had contained malignancies already. They clearly were relieved with their decision. For those women, however, who had developed breast cancer, early detection would have given them a high chance of being treated with only lumpectomy and of surviving.

Women should make the decision to have a prophylactic mastectomy with as much information as possible about the benefits and risks. Any woman considering the surgery should first try to understand why she wants to go this route. Most experts recommend that she have genetic testing to see if she's a gene mutation carrier and to see what her true risk is. She should not decide to have the surgery right after she gets the results of her genetic tests, recommends Rosenthal. "A woman who just found out she tested positive for the gene mutation won't be in the right frame of mind to make a careful decision about whether she should have the surgery done." She should also look thoroughly and carefully at the alternatives and get as much information as possible about the surveillance methods and preventive steps she can take if she decides against the surgery.

Most doctors recommend psychological counseling as well, so that a woman can make sure she's doing this for the right reasons and that she has thought through all the emotional repercussions of this procedure, says Patricia Spicer, the breast cancer program coordinator for Cancer Care, Inc., in New York. In counseling sessions, a woman can discuss her fears about breast cancer, her expectations about the surgery, what it will mean to her identity, her sense of femininity and her sexuality, and what her breasts mean to her and to her partner. She might discuss her experiences with her mother's breast cancer, and if she is grieving, she might have to work through the grief first as well. All of these emotions contribute, often unconsciously, to this decision. Partners as well as family members should be included in some discussions because the surgery will affect these relationships.

In addition to psychological and genetic counseling, any woman considering prophylactic mastectomy should get a second opinion from a doctor and also a surgical and reconstructive consultation. Taking this step is a highly individual decision with no right or wrong answer.

Still, many experts feel early detection is the answer for high-risk women. Until we can prevent breast cancer, the focus will be on preventing women from dying of breast cancer. If you follow the screening recommendations, you will improve your chances of not dying from the disease.

14

COPING

"She wanted everything to be as normal as possible, and I wanted everything to be as normal as possible, but nothing was normal."

Jenny, 24

$\mathcal{W}$hen your mother is diagnosed with breast cancer, the news can make your knees buckle or send you curling up into the fetal position to bawl. It can make you panic, as if you're in a blinding blizzard where you can only see a foot in front of you and don't know which way to turn next or how to bring yourself to safety. You may feel as if you've just been handed news of your mother's imminent death. Usually, though, you have to be strong, for it's hard to lose it in front of your mother, who needs the support and strength of her family and who is, after all, the one who is fighting for her life and who is truly suffering the most. Nonetheless, underneath that solid veneer of strength is a roiling brew of emotions to confront, emotions like disbelief and denial, fear and sadness, panic, helplessness, loss, frustration, guilt, anger, acceptance, and even grief.

Because a mother's illness threatens our sense of security in the world and because we perceive breast cancer as the disease from hell, her diagnosis can easily push the limits of our emotional endurance. But there are ways of easing the strain, coping tactics such as educating yourself about cancer and its treatments and gaining some understanding of the underlying emotional issues that make this so utterly difficult. The stories you have already read in this book dealt with many of the emotional complexities of this situation. Though nothing can take away the very real threat and the very real pain of this situation, there are ways of minimizing their burden on you.

Often the overriding feelings a daughter has at the time of her mother's diagnosis are fear for her mother's life and anxiety at seeing her so vulnerable and mortal. For most people, when they hear the word *cancer*, they fear the worst, that mother will definitely die. "In the beginning, people don't seem to take in any positive information, they don't seem to be comforted when the doctor says, 'She's going to be okay.' They don't hear anything but the word *cancer* and it's frightening," says Bruce Compas, a leading researcher of the effects of cancer on families, who works at the University of Vermont. Daughters can't help but question, "What will happen to me if mother dies?" This pessimism may persist for some time. Studies have shown that as a gender, females have a tendency to ruminate, to rehash all the possible negative outcomes of a situation. Ruminating, though, is not a very helpful coping strategy and is associated with depression, says Compas. When women are dealing with cancer, this tendency is greater because there is an element of mystery surrounding the disease—the fact that not everyone survives it, that medicine doesn't know how to cleanly and painlessly cure it leaves plenty of room for worry and pessimism. There are no absolute assurances to grasp onto.

What works far better is trying to be optimistic, though if that mode is not part of your emotional repertoire, you should at least try to be realistic. The reality of a mother's prognosis is usually a lot less grim than what daughters imagine it to be. For women diagnosed with breast cancer at an early stage, their five-year survival rate, a typical measure of the effectiveness of treatments, is 97 percent. When it's detected at Stage 1 or 2 (when cancer has spread to surrounding tissue but not other parts of the body), the five-year survival rate is 76 percent. The five-year survival rate of all women diagnosed with breast cancer when all stages are combined is still high—approximately 84 percent. Realize that for most women in whom the cancer was detected early, their families return to near emotional normalcy within six weeks. "They're going to work, not thinking about cancer incessantly, their sleeping is back to normal," says Hester Hill, manager of oncology social work at the Beth Israel Medical Center.

If you can replace your beliefs and preconceived notions of cancer with the facts, it should increase your sense of hope, or at least decrease your sense of despair. One way of doing this is to go with your mother to her doctor's appointments to hear the facts directly from the oncologist. It's easier to dismiss your mother's reassurances than the oncologist's. "If a daughter lives far away, it's helpful to visit the mother and see that she's indeed looking pretty well instead of how the daughter imagines that her mother is looking," says Hill. You should also read as much as you can. Try to educate yourself not only on survival rates but on the various cancer treatments, what your mother can expect during treatments, what follow-up care consists of, and how she can help prevent recurrences. This knowledge will help you understand that there are real steps your mother can take to survive this illness, which will help you regain a sense of control. It also takes the mystery out of the disease. It is the unknown that we tend to fear the most.

If you can take it a step further and be optimistic, this is a great self-protective coping strategy. Simply put, being optimistic is when you acknowledge that there's a problem, a dangerously steep mountain you have to climb, but you try to look on the bright side, you think of what it will be like at the top and you hope for the best, rather than feeling defeated, thinking of worst-case scenarios and being daunted by the situation. Optimism, of course, is not everyone's natural instinct, and if it's not yours, it takes time and effort to learn. If a mother deals with her illness with optimism and a fighting spirit, daughters often feel more hopeful about the outcome. On the other hand, if a mother copes with things poorly, with a sense of desperation or if she feels beaten down and falls into a depression, daughters are more likely to follow in her emotional footsteps, says UCLA psychologist David Wellisch. If you recognize this mother-daughter connection, you might be able to separate your own reaction from your mother's to better cope with your emotions.

Optimism taken to the extreme, though, is called denial—pushing onward to the top of the mountain despite the blinding blizzard that has enveloped you—and that's a coping instinct that often gets people in trouble. Trying to pretend that your mother's cancer is not a problem, that you're not at all affected by it, or trying to suppress thoughts about it doesn't work. In fact, such denials may have a rebound effect. "The harder you try to push it away, often, the more it comes back and creates fear and worry," says Compas.

Some women, in time, may come to realize that there's nothing they can do to change what has happened, and they may be able to accept the situation, or even try to find something positive in this experience, says Compas. Perhaps it has brought you and your mother closer together or has spurred some other emotional changes in you, changes in your relationships with others, or positive changes in your mother's emotional life, says Compas. Many daughters do report that the cancer has made them develop a deeper bond with their mothers. Many women with cancer say that it has made them realize what is important in their lives and has brought more meaning to their lives and to their interactions with family and friends. No one is going to say to a newly diagnosed woman or to her family that this will be a gift. It would be wrong to do so. That is something she may or may not experience, depending on her outcome, her personality, and many other factors in her life. But many women who have come down the other side of the mountain relatively healthy have used the word *gift* to describe their experience.

It can be very helpful to talk to someone about your fears for your mother's life, either a therapist, social worker, or other professional. If that's not possible, then talking to close family members, your partner or spouse, or your close friends can help, too. Allowing yourself to verbalize your fears and to share your concerns with others usually leaves you feeling lighter. Indeed, it is an important part of the healing process. Your confidants may even surprise you with some sound advice or may share with you a similar experience they've had, or at least they'll be able to offer some hands-on support in the day-to-day demands of dealing with a sick mother. Likewise, releasing your fears through writing may also be productive.

When women are given a good prognosis, typically their families feel in crisis for a period of around six to eight weeks, says Hill. If you find you have fairly intense emotions and are obsessed about her dying for much longer than that, despite your mother's good prognosis, you may need to go for counseling, Hill advises. "The goal for every woman and her family," says Hill, "is to live as if the cancer isn't going to come back, because living any other way just wrecks your life."

If your mother's prognosis is not good, if she is going to be getting sicker and increasingly disabled, that's a good reason to be feeling distressed, fearful, angry, and depressed. When cancer metastasizes to other organs, it's as if the family's whole world changes. Hope and high survival rates are replaced with onerous treatments and less encouraging statistics, even though many women do live years after their cancer has metastasized. Life becomes more of a roller-coaster ride, as each doctor's visit brings new news—a positive report one month, a negative report the next. First, "Everything looks clean on the CAT scan." Then, "We see a shadow." It goes back and forth, and during that time, you may alternate between holding out hope and beginning to grieve. "The bottom line is that if your mother is dying, it's one of the worst things that happens to you in life," says Hill. There's no easy way to cope because there's no way to make the situation go away. This is a time when you need to talk about your feelings with others. You need to talk about your fears and your losses. You have already lost not your mother, but your healthy mother, the one who was vivacious and helpful and reprimanding and supportive and keenly interested in your life. A woman battered by repeated cancer treatments does not have the energy to fulfill her motherly roles.

One of the most difficult and stressful things for daughters is to reverse roles and provide their mothers with emotional and physical support during their illness. Women often find themselves in the role of caregivers during difficult times, which does not come without a cost to them. It is difficult on both emotional and practical fronts. Emotionally, this is a role reversal that many young women are not ready for. It makes women face the fact that their mother is not there for them. "The mother is focused on her own health and her own survival and the changes to her body, and the daughter has to come to grips with the loss of her mother's full attention. And now she has to turn her own attention from herself too, and to her mother," says Roberta Hufnagel, a New York City psychotherapist who works with breast cancer patients and their daughters. Younger women who were living a carefree life up until this point suddenly have to become super responsible and give up the freedom of youth. Even children are called upon to take on more responsibilities and become little moms. Another difficulty for caretaking daughters is that they are continually exposed to their mother's failing health. If a woman's health and body are deteriorating, and a daughter is tending to her on a day-to-day basis, it's a constant and devastating reminder of her mother's mortality and her mother's fate. Moreover, daughters report that seeing their mother in pain is one of the most difficult things they have had to endure.

Practically, becoming the caretaker can deplete your own resources. You may be able to keep it up for a short time, but eventually you may become exhausted and overburdened. Some women feel that they have to give everything they have, every minute that isn't occupied by their work, and some even feel they have to leave their jobs or leave their own families to take care of their mothers. If your mother is dying and you know time is short, this may be appropriate, but if your mother needs caretaking over the long run, this may be too much of a sacrifice.

"It's really important, if the daughter is there helping with the care, to remember that you still have to take charge of your own life. You still have a life and you still have to pay attention to it and not let mother's illness take center stage," says Hill. Mental health professionals like to spell out caretakers' rights, because some patients or other family members may expect you to do the unreasonable, and some patients may try to manipulate you with guilt or depression. Caregivers have the right to take care of their own needs and maintain the other facets of their life. You should not be expected or expect yourself to drop everything in your life. Try to maintain your own physical health, try to exercise, which can be a great release of stress. Even though you may feel selfish tending to your own needs, it's an important way for you to keep your sanity. This in turn will allow you to be a better caretaker to your mother. If you begin to feel consistently resentful and too self-sacrificing, you need to find other solutions, or else you'll end up feeling bitter and hostile, says psychologist Evelyn Bassoff of Boulder, Colorado. Likewise, don't expect to always be patient and loving. You may get annoyed with your mother and frustrated at times. It is important and okay to recognize your personal limitations. There is not an appropriate amount of time you should spend with your mother; it's what you're capable of. Everyone has a different threshold. "Someone who feels guilty that she's not there enough, but she can't handle being there any more than she is, has to see her own limitations and make her mother recognize them as well," says Kash.

One of the solutions to feeling overextended is asking others to help. Caretakers have the right to ask family and friends for help. The first person to look toward is your father if he is not participating enough in the physical caretaking. Some men may naturally step aside and let their daughters do this type of providing. Working outside the home may make it difficult for some fathers to chip in, and some abandon the process altogether to the daughter, says Wellisch. To get a father involved, inform him of the toll it's taking on you and ask him to help.

Don't be afraid to reach out to other family members, siblings, aunts, uncles, and cousins, or even your mother's friends. Don't wait for them to ask if you need any help. If you have your own close friends, they may be able to help you manage things in your life that have fallen through the cracks during your mother's illness, or they may be able to take on some responsibilities like driving your children to afterschool activities when you're busy with your mother or watching your children for an afternoon. Don't be afraid to take up friends' offers of help, even if you think you can handle it all yourself. Usually these are not idle offers. Good friends genuinely want to help you through this but often don't know what to say or do for you. If it's necessary, you also have the right to get outside help from an organization like Cancer Care or by hiring a nurse. Check into community and national resources (see *Resources*). If your mother or another relative objects to your turning to outside help, you have the right to assert your own limits by explaining that this is a necessary step to take.

Though you may feel that you need to be emotionally

strong for your mother, it's okay to show and express your feelings to her, whether anger, sadness, hopelessness, or fear. Remember that your feelings, however ugly they may seem to you, are normal. Having these emotions isn't going to change the course of your mother's illness for better or worse. Even if they may hurt her or make her feel guilty that you're suffering too, often confiding feelings brings mothers and daughters much closer together than if they kept the feelings to themselves for fear of burdening the other.

You'll definitely want to reward yourself once in a while for the effort you have made on your mother's behalf. You may feel that it was a no-brainer to be there for your mother, but that doesn't take away from the fact that it's a difficult, tremendous responsibility.

Fear for Yourself

Once a mother's situation stabilizes, it's common for a daughter to begin to fear for her own life. The level of anxiety daughters feel often corresponds to how well or poorly their mother fared and whether she survived. If a mother dies, it dramatically raises the daughter's fear for herself, and the grief also adds to the intensity of the emotions she has to cope with. Watching a mother suffer and ultimately die of cancer may create post-traumatic stress if the experience during her illness was horrifying to the daughter, and this can heighten all of a daughter's feelings, including her fear for her own life. Many daughters who have seen their mothers die a painful death fear dying the same terrifying way.

There are several ways of dealing with the fear of cancer. The first is talking about the experience of your mother's illness and if she died, talking about her death. Speaking with a professional psychologist or counselor or simply a friend can help you work through some of your fears, your sadness, your losses, and your grief, which in turn may ease your fears. Many women are surprised at the feelings that surface once they begin to retell the experience. If you are grieving, try to join a bereavement group, because sharing your feelings with others who are grieving has been shown to ease the pain and help move people through the grieving process.

Next, begin to take back control of your life. "A lot of women come in with a sense of doom and powerlessness against cancer. They feel like the cancer is in their families, therefore it's in their genes and there's nothing they can do about it," says Kash. But as you've seen in previous chapters, educating yourself on your risks and on the prevention tactics and the realities of cancer will in most instances decrease your anxiety. The less anxious you are, the more likely you'll be to follow the recommendations for breast exams and mammography or to make some lifestyle changes—losing weight or cutting back on alcohol—that may reduce your risks. The cycle perpetuates itself. The more you follow the recommendations, the less anxious you'll feel. When you're doing all the right things, self-exams, breast exams, and mammography, not only do you feel that you've taken control of your life, but you increase your chances of catching a cancer early and surviving it with the least trauma to your body. That can be reassuring. Having a good doctor who takes you seriously and a good place to get mammograms can also ease anxiety for daughters, says Margaret Burke, social work supervisor at Cancer Care. If you feel that your doctor is not on top of things or is not aggressive enough with your surveillance program, then look for a better doctor or cancer prevention center.

It also helps to talk to others about your fears, but in this case, it may be most helpful to talk to other daughters. Currently, there are very few support groups for daughters of women with breast cancer around the country. That is a problem. There is the need, but it is a silent need. Daughters need to inquire about groups at their local cancer prevention centers and nonprofit cancer organizations. If enough daughters demand support groups, these organizations will recognize the need and will consider starting groups for daughters. In the future, support groups for children of cancer patients may be as common as support groups for cancer patients and for their spouses.

Aside from cancer-specific tactics, try to use ways of coping that have worked for you in the past. Some effective tactics include exercise, progressive relaxation techniques, yoga and meditation, or even gardening, baking, or any other hobby you enjoy. There's a tendency to consider these activities frivolous pursuits during this period of hardship when extra demands are made on your time, but they can help you stay calm, maintain an even keel, and have some semblance of balance in your life. It's okay, and actually healthy, to try to eke out some enjoyment of life, even when your mother is facing cancer. Women who seem to fare well have learned to bring a sense of humor to their situations and not take every little thing as a sign of doom.

What can also be helpful for daughters is volunteering for the breast cancer cause. Taking action is one of the best ways to overcome feelings of helplessness and fear, says Wellisch. Doing advocacy work for breast cancer organizations or trying to raise money for the cause through events such as the Race for the Cure can also make you feel that you're doing something for your own future, because you're participating in the fight to get better treatments and find a better, kinder cure for cancer. Likewise, being exposed to women in these groups, who are for the most part survivors of breast cancer, can bring you hope for your situation and your future, even if that future has a diagnosis of breast cancer. If your mother has died from cancer, it can be especially helpful to expose yourself to survivors so that you can see firsthand that there are other ways that cancer can turn out, other than in death. Survivors, by dint of what they have experienced, are typically strong, inspiring, incredible women, and they will without a doubt fill you with hope.

NOTES

p. 4 The statistics on breast cancer are from the American Cancer Society, *Cancer Facts & Figures*.

p. 4 *"daughters do tend to have more intrusive thoughts"* C. Lerman, K. Kash, M. Stefanek, "Younger Women at Increased Risk for Breast Cancer: Perceived Risk, Psychological Well-being, and Surveillance Behavior," *Journal of the National Cancer Institute Monographs* 1994, 16:171.

p. 4 *"Compas's studies conclude"* E. K. Grant, B. E. Compas, "Stress and Anxious-Depressed Symptoms Among Adolescents: Searching for Mechanisms of Risk," *Journal of Consulting and Clinical Psychology* 1995, 63(6):1015.

p. 6 *"David Wellisch found that when a mother dies"* D. K. Wellisch, E. R. Gritz, W. Schain, et al., "Psychological Functioning of Daughters of Breast Cancer Patients," (Part 1), *Psychosomatics* 1991, 32:324; (Part 2), *Psychosomatics* 1992, 33:171.

p. 26 *"Jungian book"* K. Carlson, *In Her Image: The Unhealed Daughter's Search for Her Mother*, Boston & London: Shambhala, 1990.

p. 39 *"This increase in their responsibilities"* Grant & Compas, 1995.

p. 67 *"a study by Frances Marcus Lewis"* E. H. Zahlis, F. M. Lewis, "The Mother's Story of the School-Age Child's Experience with the Mother's Breast Cancer," *Journal of Psychosocial Oncology*. In press.

p. 139 *"according to a study of high-risk women"* Lerman, Kash, & Stefanek, 1994.

p. 141 *"Though estimates vary, only 6 to 19 percent"* K. F. Hoskins, J. E. Stopfer, et al., "Assessment and Counseling for Women with a Family History of Breast Cancer," *Journal of the American Medical Association* 1995, 273(7):577.

p. 142 *"women who had high levels of anxiety"* C. Lerman, E. Lustbader, et al., "Effects of Individualized Breast Cancer Risk Counseling: A Randomized Trial," *Journal of the National Cancer Institute* 1995, 87(4):286.

p. 146 *"Stopfer and her coauthors divided women into two at-risk groups"* Hoskins, Stopfer, et al., 1995.

p. 151 *"Indeed, the American Cancer Society (ACS)"* Statement of the American Society of Human Genetics on genetic testing for breast and ovarian cancer predisposition, *American Journal of Genetics* 1994, 55:i.

p. 152 *"Studies show that when high-risk women are given the option"* C. Lerman, M. D. Schwartz, S. Narod, H. T. Lynch, "The Influence of Psychological Distress on Use of Genetic Testing for Cancer Risk," *Journal of Consulting and Clinical Psychology* 1997, 65(3):414.

p. 152 *"Those who are more likely to get tested"* Lerman, Schwartz, Narod, & Lynch, 1997.

p. 155 *"At the state level"* National Cancer Institute: State Cancer Legislative Database Program 1998.

p. 155 *"In a study of depression in high-risk women"* C. Lerman, C. Hughes, et al., "What You Don't Know Can Hurt You: Adverse Psychologic Effects in Members of BRCA1-Linked and BRCA2-Linked Families Who Decline Genetic Testing," *Journal of Clinical Oncology* 1998, 16(5):1650.

p. 156 *"In anxious women who turned down the test"* Lerman, Hughes, et al., 1998.

p. 160 *"a direct correlation between fear and screening behaviors"* K. M. Kash, "Psychosocial and Ethical Implications of Defining Genetic Risk for Cancers," *Annals of the New York Academy of Sciences* 1995, 768:41.

p. 161 *"Several clinical trials have found that regular screening mammography"* R. E. Hendrick, R. A. Smith, J. H. Rutledge, C. R. Smart, "Benefit of Screening Mammography in Women Aged 40–49: A New Meta-Analysis of Randomized Controlled Trials," *Journal of the National Cancer Institute Monographs* 1997, 22:87.

p. 161 *"There certainly is a need for early detection"* American Cancer Society: Breast Cancer Facts and Figures 1996, American Cancer Society, Atlanta Ga., 1996.

p. 161 *"tumors detected by mammographic screening"* Hendrick, Smith, Rutledge, & Smart, 1997.

p. 161 *"Mammograms miss up to 25 percent"* NIH Consensus Statement Breast Cancer Screening for Women Ages 40–49, 1997.

p. 162 *"For every eight biopsies"* NIH Consensus Statement Breast Cancer Screening for Women Ages 40–49, 1997.

p. 162 *"a 29 percent reduction"* Hendrick, Smith, Rutledge, & Smart, 1997.

p. 162 *"They recommend annual mammography"* W. Burke et al. for the Cancer Genetics Studies Consortium. "Recommendations for Follow-up Care of Individuals with an Inherited Predisposition to Cancer," *Journal of the American Medical Association* 1997, 277(12):997.

p. 163 *"Ten percent of breast cancers"* Burke et al., 1997.

p. 163 *"For women with a family history"* Burke et al., 1997.

p. 164 *"Monthly BSE is recommended"* Burke et al., 1997.

p. 165 *"A meta-analysis of data from fifty-four studies"* Collaborative

Group on Hormonal Factors in Breast Cancer, "Breast Cancer and Hormonal Contraceptives," *Lancet* 1996, 347:1713.

p. 166 *"This reduction in risk after ten years"* Collaborative Group on Hormonal Factors, 1996.

p. 166 *"women who started birth control pills early in life"* E. White, K. E. Malone, N. S. Weiss, J. R. Daling, "Breast Cancer Among Young U.S. Women in Relation to Oral Contraceptive Use," *Journal of the National Cancer Institute* 1994, 86(7):505.

p. 166 *"a reduced risk—as much as 60 percent"* S. A. Narod, H. Risch, R. Moslehi, et al., "Oral Contraceptives and the Risk of Hereditary Ovarian Cancer," *New England Journal of Medicine* 1998, 339(7):424.

p. 166 *"A 1995 study conducted by Kent Hoskins"* Hoskins, Stopfer, et al., 1995.

p. 167 *"about 25 percent of women who reach menopause"* M. Porter, G. C. Penney, et al., "A Population-Based Survey of Women's Experience of the Menopause," *British Journal of Obstetrics and Gynaecology* 1996, 103:1025.

p. 167 *"HRT has also been recommended to women"* E. Barrett-Connor, D. Grady, "Hormone Replacement Therapy, Heart Disease, and Other Considerations," *Annual Review of Public Health* 1998, 19:55.

p. 167 *"This bias in the study population"* G. A. Colditz, "Relationship between Estrogen Levels, Use of Hormone Replacement Therapy, and Breast Cancer," *Journal of the National Cancer Institute* 1998, 90(11):814.

p. 168 *"For those who had taken estrogen for five years or longer"* Collaborative Group on Hormonal Factors in Breast Cancer, "Breast Cancer and Hormone Replacement Therapy: Combined Reanalysis of Data from 51 Epidemiological Studies," *Lancet* 1997, 350:1047.

p. 168 *"breast cancer risk returns to that of the general population"* C. W. Burger, N. A. Koomen, et al., "Postmenopausal Hormone Replacement Therapy and Cancer of the Female Genital Tract and the Breast," *European Menopause Journal* 1997, 4(1):22.

p. 168 *"The risk seems to be higher for overweight women"* A. Huang, S. E. Hankinson, G. A. Colditz, et al., "Dual Effects of Weight and Weight Gain on Breast Cancer Risk," *Journal of the American Medical Association* 1997, 278(17):1407.

p. 169 *"The study also concluded that weight gain"* Huang, Hankinson, Colditz, et al., 1997.

p. 169 *"When premenopausal women were examined alone"* I. Thune, T. Brenn, E. Lunde, M. Gaard, "Physical Activity and the Risk of Breast Cancer," *New England Journal of Medicine* 1997, 336(18):1269.

p. 169 *"An analysis of the exercise habits of more than 100,000 women"* B. Rockhill, W. C. Willett, E. Hunter, et al., "Physical Activity and Breast Cancer Risk in a Cohort of Young Women," *Journal of the National Cancer Institute* 1998, 90(15):155.

p. 170 *"Although there's no good explanation for how fat"* J. R. Harris, M. E. Lippman, U. Veronesi, W. Willett, "Breast Cancer," *New England Journal of Medicine* 1992, 327(5):319.

p. 171 *"Experts recommend lowering fat intake"* E. L. Wydner, "Reflections on Diet, Nutrition, and Cancer," *Cancer Research* 1983, 43:3024.

p. 171 *"Compared with nondrinkers"* S. A. Smith-Warner, D. Spiegelman, et al., "Alcohol and Breast Cancer in Women: A Pooled Analysis of Cohort Studies," *Journal of the American Medical Association* 1998, 279(7):535.

p. 172 *"results from the Breast Cancer Prevention Trial"* B. Fisher, J. P. Costantino, et al., "Tamoxifen for Prevention of Breast Cancer: Report of the National Surgical Adjuvant Breast and Bowel Project P-1 Study," *Journal of the National Cancer Institute* 1998, 90(18):1371.

p. 173 *"An analysis of 7,705 women"* Preliminary results from the ongoing Multiple Outcomes of Raloxifene Evaluation study, announced at the annual meeting of the European Congress on Osteoporosis, Berlin, Germany 1998.

p. 174 *"A 1997 consensus paper"* Burke et al., 1997.

p. 175 *"A 1999 Study"* L. Hartmann, et al., "Efficacy of Bilateral Prophylactic Mastectomy in Women with a Family History of Breast Cancer," *The New England Journal of Medicine* 1999, 340:77.

p. 180 *"females have a tendency to ruminate"* Grant & Compas, 1995.

p. 184 *"Younger women who were living a carefree life"* B. E. Compas, N. L. Worsham, et al., "When Mom or Dad Has Cancer: Markers of Psychological Distress in Cancer Patients, Spouses, and Children," *Health Psychology* 1994, 13(6):507.

RESOURCES

General Information

Organizations offering general information on breast cancer, risk, prevention, and support:

American Cancer Society
1599 Clifton Road, NE
Atlanta, GA 30329
800-ACS-2345
Web site: http://www.cancer.org
A nationwide, community-based organization with chartered divisions in each state. ACS focuses on research and education but also provides patient services, family support groups, caregiver counseling, and cancer information.

Cancer Care, Inc.
1180 Avenue of the Americas
New York, NY 10036
800-813-HOPE
212-302-2400
Web site: http://www.cancercareinc.org
A social service agency that provides professional counseling, financial assistance, insurance counseling, support groups, workshops, teleconferences, telephone, and on-line support groups for women with cancer, their family members, and caregivers.

Gilda Radner Familial Ovarian Cancer Registry
Roswell Park Cancer Institute
Elm and Carlton Street
Buffalo, NY 14263
800-OVA-RIAN
Collects data on the link between heredity and ovarian can-
cer. Also provides general counseling, support groups, and assis-
tance with genetic screening.

Hereditary Cancer Institute
Creighten University School of Medicine
California at 24th Street
Omaha, NE 68178
800-648-8133
402-280-2942
Studies hereditary cancer and offers counseling and information about clinical trials for women with cancer and their
families.

National Alliance of Breast Cancer Organizations
(NABCO)
9 East 37th Street, 10th Floor
New York, NY 10016
212-889-0606
800-719-9154 (outside NYC)
web site: http://www.nabco.org
A network of breast cancer organizations that provides
information, assistance, and referral about breast cancer and acts
as a voice for the interests and concerns of breast cancer survivors and women at risk.

National Cancer Institute
800-4-CANCER
web site: http://cancernet.nci.nih.gov
The U.S. agency responsible for conducting and supporting
research on cancer. Services include the Physicians Data Query
(PDQ), a computerized listing of cancer information and
resources, a nationwide hotline, and a fax information retrieval
system.

National Family Caregivers Association
9621 East Bexhill Drive
Kensington, MD 20895
800-896-3650
301-942-6430
web site: http://www.nfcacares.org
Provides research, education support, respite care, and advocacy for caregivers.

SHARE
1501 Broadway, 17th Floor
New York, NY 10036
212-382-2111 (hotline)
A self-help organization that offers information and support groups for women with breast or ovarian cancer and their families.

Sisters Network, Inc.
8787 Woodway Drive
Suite 4207
Houston, TX 77063
713-781-0255
Provides information and support groups for African American women with breast cancer.

Susan G. Komen Breast Cancer Foundation
3500 Gaston Sammons Tower No. 320
Dallas, TX 75246
800-IM-AWARE
214-450-1777
Web site: http://www.komen.org
An organization that funds research, provides breast cancer news and information and referrals to support groups, and sponsors the Race for the Cure. Many local chapters.

Celebrating Life Foundation
P.O. Box 224076
Dallas, TX 75222-4076
800-207-0992

web site: http://www.celebratinglife.org
Promotes breast cancer awareness, specifically targeting African American women and women of color.

Wellness Community
2716 Ocean Park Boulevard, Suite 1040
Santa Monica, CA 90405
310-314-2555
Wellness communities provide free psychosocial support to people recovering from cancer and their families. There are fourteen Wellness Community facilities nationwide.

Y-Me National Breast Cancer Organization
212 West Van Buren Street, 4th Floor
Chicago, IL 60607
800-221-2141
800-986-9505 (Spanish)
312-986-8228
Web site: http://y-me.org
Provides information and support to women with breast cancer and their families and friends through a national hotline, open door groups, and early detection workshops. Y-Me has many local chapters.

Early Detection Resources

BSE Shower Card. Two groups offer a waterproof shower card guide to breast self-examination. For one free card, write to AMC Cancer Research Center, Marketing and Public Relations Department, 1600 Pierce Street, Denver, CO 80214, 800-321-1557, or 303-233-6501 in Colorado. Or call the American Cancer Society, 800-ACS-2345.

How to do BSE. A pamphlet provided by the American Cancer Society that offers specific instructions on breast self-examination. 800-ACS-2345.

Getting the Best Mammogram. This one-page NABCO fact sheet gives advice on getting a quality mammogram. Call 888-80-NABCO.

Understanding Breast Changes: A Health Guide for All Women (96-3536). This booklet explains various types of breast changes that women experience and describes diagnostic tests that distinguish between benign changes and cancer. Call NCI at 800-4-CANCER.

Risk Counseling and Testing

Genetic Testing for Cancer Risk: It's Your Choice. A video providing an overview of the risk and benefits of being tested for genetic mutation. Brochure available too. Write to National Action Plan on Breast Cancer, PHS Office on Women's Health, 200 Independence Ave. SW, Room 718F, Washington, DC 20201.

Understanding Genetics of Breast Cancer for Jewish Women. This brochure answers questions about hereditary risk of breast cancer and whether genetic testing is appropriate for you. Available by calling the Hadassah Health Education Department at 212-303-8094.

Understanding Gene Testing (96-3905). This brochure provides basic information about genetic mutations and testing and addresses the concerns of someone considering testing under the current state of managed care. Call the NCI at 800-4-CANCER.

Genetic Counselors

The National Cancer Institute provides a directory of genetic counselors on its web site: http://cancernet.nci.nih.gov/www-prot/genetic/background.html

National Society of Genetic Counselors, Inc., provides a directory of genetic counselors. Call, write, or check their Internet site:
NSGC
233 Canterbury Drive
Wallingford, PA 19086.
610-872-7608.
web site: http://www.nsgc.org

Breast Cancer Advocacy

National Breast Cancer Coalition
1707 L Street, NW, Suite 1060
Washington, DC 20036
202-296-7477
Web site: http://www.natlbcc.org
A grassroots organization formed to eradicate breast cancer through action and advocacy by increasing research funding and access of medical care to all women, and bringing breast cancer to the forefront of the nation's agenda.

Community Breast Health Project
545 Bryant Street
Palo Alto, CA 94301
650-326-6686
web site: http://www-med.stanford.edu/CBHP
A clearinghouse for information and support, providing volunteer opportunities for breast cancer survivors and friends dedicated to helping others with the disease, and serving as an educational resource about breast cancer and breast health.

Information on breast cancer legislation can be found on the web site:
http://members.aol.com/BCLegis/index.htm

Comprehensive Cancer Centers

A state by state list of centers that offer screening, risk counseling, and follow-up for high-isk women.
For additional listings, the National Consortium of Breast Centers offers referrals to centers nationwide. When you call, ask specifically for centers that offer services to high-risk women.

National Consortium of Breast Centers
P.O. Box 1334
Warsaw, IN 46581
219-267-8058
e-mail: wiggins@breastcare.org
web site: http://breastcare.org

ALABAMA
UAB Comprehensive Cancer Center
University of Alabama at Birmingham
1824 Sixth Avenue South
Birmingham, AL 35293-3300
205-934-5077
web site: http://www.ccc.uab.edu

ARIZONA
Arizona Cancer Center
University of Arizona
1501 North Campbell Avenue
Tucson, AZ 85724
520-626-6044
web site: http://www.azcc.arizona.edu

CALIFORNIA
Alta Bates-Herrick Comprehensive Cancer Center
Herrick Campus
2001 Dwight Way
Berkeley, CA 94704
510-204-1591
web site: http://www.altabates.com

City of Hope National Medical Center
1500 East Duarte Road
Duarte, CA 91010-3000
626-359-8111
web site: http://www.cityofhope.org

Stanford University Medical Center
Division of Oncology
Stanford, CA 94305-5515
650-723-7621

UCSD Cancer Center
University of California at San Diego
9500 Gilman Drive
La Jolla, CA 92093-0658
619-534-7600
web site: http://cancer.ucsd.edu/

Jonsson Comprehensive Cancer Center
University of California, Los Angeles
Factor Bldg., Room 8-684
10833 Le Conte Avenue
Los Angeles, CA 90095-1781
310-825-5268 or 800-825-2144
web site: http://www.cancer.mednet.ucla.edu

USC/Norris Comprehensive Cancer Center
University of Southern California
1441 Eastlake Avenue
Los Angeles, CA 90033
323-865-3371
web site: http://ccnt.hsc.usc.edu

Chao Family Comprehensive Cancer Center
University of California at Irvine
101 City Drive, Bldg. 23
Rt. 81, Room 406
Orange, CA 92868
714-456-8030
web site: http://www.ucihs.uci.edu/cancer/

COLORADO
University of Colorado Cancer Center
University of Colorado Health Science Center
4200 East 9th Avenue, Box B188
Denver, CO 80262
303-315-3007
web site:
http://www.uchsc.edu/chancllr/UCCC/UCCCwelcome.html

CONNECTICUT
Yale Cancer Center
Yale University School of Medicine
333 Cedar Street, Box 208028
New Haven, CT 06520-8028
203-785-4095
web site: http://www.info.med.yale.edu/ycc

DISTRICT OF COLUMBIA
Lombardi Cancer Research Center
Georgetown University Medical Center
3800 Reservoir Road, NW
Washington, DC 20007
202-687-2192
web site: http://lombardi.georgetown.edu

FLORIDA
H. Lee Moffitt Cancer Center & Research Institute
University of South Florida
12902 Magnolia Drive
Tampa, FL 33612-9497
813-972-4673
web site: http://www.moffitt.usf.edu

Comprehensive Cancer Center
4306 Alton Road
Miami Beach, FL 33140
305-535-3434

Comprehensive Cancer Center at JFK Medical Center
5301 South Congress Avenue
Atlantis, FL 33462
561-964-2662
web site: http://www.jfkmc.com/cancer_center.htm

HAWAII
Cancer Research Center of Hawaii
University of Hawaii at Manoa
1236 Lauhala Street
Honolulu, HI 96813
808-586-3010
web site: http://www2.hawaii.edu/crch

ILLINOIS
Cancer Research Center
University of Chicago Cancer Research Center
5841 South Maryland Avenue, MC 1140
Chicago, IL 60637-1470
773-702-9200
web site: http://www-uccrc.bsd.uchicago.edu

Lynn Sage Comprehensive Breast Center
Northwestern Memorial Hospital
333 East Superior Street
Chicago, IL 60611
312-908-8822

MARYLAND
Johns Hopkins Breast Center
600 North Wolfe Street, Room 157
Baltimore, MD 21287-8943
410-955-4851
web site: http://ww2.med.jhu.edu/cancerctr

MASSACHUSETTS
Cancer Center
Dana-Farber Cancer Institute
44 Binney Street, Room 1828
Boston, MA 02115
617-632-3000
web site: http://www.dfci.harvard.edu

MICHIGAN
Comprehensive Cancer Center
University of Michigan 6302, CGC/0942
1500 East Medical Center Drive
Ann Arbor, MI 48l09-0942
734-647-8900
web site: http://www.cancer.med.umich.edu

Barbara Ann Karmanos Cancer Institute
Wayne State University
   operating the Meyer L. Prentis Comprehensive Cancer
   Center of Metropolitan Detroit
4100 John R. Street
Detroit, MI 48201-1379
800-527-6266
web site: http://www.karmanos.org

MINNESOTA
Cancer Center
University of Minnesota
Box 806
420 Delaware Street, SE
Minneapolis, MN 55455
612-624-8484
web site: http://www.cancer.umn.edu

Mayo Cancer Center
Mayo Clinic
200 First Street, SW
Rochester, MN 55905
507-284-2511

NEBRASKA
Eppley Cancer Center
University of Nebraska Medical Center
Omaha, NE
402-559-4090
web site: http://www.unmc.edu

NEW HAMPSHIRE
Norris Cotton Cancer Center
Dartmouth-Hitchcock Medical Center
One Medical Center Drive
Hinman Box 7920
Lebanon, NH 03756-0001
603-650-6300
web site: http://NCCC.hitchcock.org

NEW JERSEY
Cancer Institute of New Jersey
Robert Wood Johnson Medical School
195 Little Albany Street, Room 2002B
New Brunswick, NJ 08901
732-235-6777
web site: http://130.219.231.104

NEW YORK
Cancer Research Center
Albert Einstein College of Medicine
Chanin Bldg., Room 209
1300 Morris Park Avenue
Bronx, NY 10461
718-430-2302
web site: http://www.ca.aecom.yu.edu

Roswell Park Cancer Institute
Elm & Carlton Streets
Buffalo, NY 14263-0001
716-845-2300 or 800-Roswell
web site: http://rpci.med.buffalo.edu

Kaplan Cancer Center
New York University Medical Center
550 First Avenue
New York, NY 10016
212-263-5343
web site: http://kccc-www.med.nyu.edu/

Special Surveillance Breast Program
Memorial Sloan-Kettering Cancer Center
1275 York Avenue
New York, NY 10021
212-639-5250 or 800-525-2225
web site: http://www.mskcc.org

Strang Cancer Prevention Center
428 East 72nd Street
New York, NY 10021
212-794-4900
web site: http://www.strang.org

Herbert Irving Comprehensive Cancer Center
Columbia University
161 Fort Washington Avenue
10th Floor
New York, NY 10032
212-326-8550
web site: http://www.ccc.columbia.edu
Also contact Columbia's Women at Risk program:
    212-305-9525

University of Rochester Cancer Center
601 Elmwood Avenue
Rochester, NY 14642
716-275-4911
web site:
http://www.urmc.rochester.edu/strong/cancer

NORTH CAROLINA
UNC Lineberger Comprehensive Cancer Center
University of North Carolina, Chapel Hill
School of Medicine, CB-7295
Chapel Hill, NC 27599-7295
919-966-3036
web site: http://www.med.unc.edu/wrkunits/3ctrpgm/lccc

Duke Comprehensive Cancer Center
Duke University Medical Center
Box 3843
Durham, NC 27710
919-684-5613
web site: http://www.canctr.mc.duke.edu

Comprehensive Cancer Center
Wake Forest University
Bowman Gray School of Medicine
Medical Center Boulevard
Winston-Salem, NC 27157-1082
336-716-7971
web site: http://www.bgsm.edu/cancer

OHIO
Ireland Cancer Center
Case Western Reserve University and University Hospitals
    of Cleveland
11100 Euclid Avenue
Cleveland, OH 44106-5065
216-844-5432 or 800-641-2422
web site: http://www.uhhs.com/uhc/cancer/index.html

Comprehensive Cancer Center
Arthur G. James Cancer Hospital
Ohio State University
A455 Staring Loving Hall
300 West 10th Avenue
Columbus, OH 43210-1240
614-293-3300
web site: http://www-cancer.med.ohio-state.edu

OREGON
Oregon Cancer Center
Oregon Health Sciences University
3181 SW Sam Jackson Park Road
Portland, OR 97201-3098
503-494-1617
web site: http://www.ohsu.edu

PENNSYLVANIA
University of Pennsylvania Cancer Center
Penn Tower
3401 Civic Center Boulevard
Philadelphia, PA 19104-4283
215-349-8382
web site: http://cancer.med.upenn.edu

Fox Chase Cancer Center
7701 Burholme Avenue
Philadelphia, PA 19111
215-728-6900
web site: http://www.fccc.edu

Kimmel Cancer Center
Thomas Jefferson Hospital
111 South 11th Street
BLSB, Room 1050
Philadelphia, PA 19107
800-JEFF-NOW
web site: http://morrison.jci.tju.edu

Comprehensive Breast Care Center
University of Pittsburgh Cancer Institute
UPMC Montefiore, 7 Main
200 Lothrop Street
Pittsburgh, PA 15213-3305
800-237-4724
web site: http://www.pci.upmc.edu

TENNESSEE
Breast Center
Vanderbilt University
1500 21st Avenue South
Nashville, TN 37212
615-322-2064 or 800-811-8480
web site: http://www.mc.vanderbilt.edu/vumc/centers/
    cancer.html

TEXAS
Cancer Prevention Center
University of Texas M.D. Anderson Cancer Center
1515 Holcombe Boulevard
Houston, TX 77030
713-745-8040 or 800-438-6434
web site: http://www.mdanderson.org

San Antonio Cancer Institute
8122 Datapoint Drive, Suite 600
San Antonio, TX 78229-3264
210-616-5500
web site: http://www.ccc.saci.org

University of Texas Southwestern Center for Breast Care
James W. Aston Ambulatory Care Center
5323 Harry Hines Boulevard
Dallas, TX 75235
214-648-8969

UTAH
Huntsman Cancer Institute
University of Utah
15 North 2030 East
Salt Lake City, UT 84112
801-581-6365 or 888-424-2100
web site: http://www.hci.utah.edu

VERMONT
Vermont Cancer Center
One South Prospect Street
Burlington, VT 05401
802-656-4414
web site: http//www.vtmednet.org/vcc

VIRGINIA
Cancer Center
University of Virginia, Health Sciences Center Hospital
Box 334
Charlottesville, VA 22908
804-924-3627 or 800-251-3627
web site: http://www.med.virginia.edu/medcntr/cancer

Massey Cancer Center
Virginia Commonwealth University
401 College Street
Richmond, VA 23298
804-828-0450
web site: http://views.vcu.edu/mcc

WASHINGTON
Fred Hutchinson Cancer Research Center
1100 Fairview Avenue, North
Seattle, WA 98109
206-667-5000
web site: http://www.fhcrc.org

WISCONSIN
Comprehensive Cancer Center
University of Wisconsin
600 Highland Avenue, Room K4-6
Madison, WI 53792
608-263-8600
web site: http://www.medsch.wisc.edu/cancer/homepage

GLOSSARY

adenocarcinoma—Cancer that starts in glandular tissue— the ducts or lobules of the breast. Most breast cancers are adenocarcinomas.

Adriamycin—One of several drugs used during chemotherapy.

advanced cancer—Typically describes a stage in which the cancer has spread to other parts of the body. Locally advanced cancer means the cancer has spread only to the surrounding area. Metastatic cancer means it has spread, through the bloodstream or lymphatic system, to other organs in the body.

anovulation—When ovulation does not occur and a woman doesn't have her period.

antiestrogen—A substance that blocks the effects of estrogen on tumors by attaching to the tumor cells' estrogen receptors. Antiestrogens, like the drug tamoxifen, are used to treat breast cancers that depend on estrogen for growth, and preventively to reduce the chances of cancers developing.

atypical hyperplasia—An abnormal increase in the number of atypical or irregular cells in a specific area, such as the lining of the breast ducts or the lobules. Atypical hyperplasia can increase the risk of a cancer developing.

benign—Not cancerous.

biopsy—The removal of a tissue sample for examination under a microscope to find out if cancer or other abnormal cells are present. A biopsy can be done with a needle, which draws out a sample from a suspicious lump, or by surgery, which typically removes an entire lump.

bone marrow transplant (BMT)—The term *bone marrow transplant* has been replaced by the term *stem cell transplant,* which more accurately describes this procedure. (See stem cell transplant)

BRCA1 & BRCA2—Acronyms for Breast Cancer genes 1 and 2. If someone has inherited a damaged or mutated BRCA gene, she is at a much higher risk of developing breast cancer and ovarian cancer than the average population. The BRCA genes are cancer suppressor genes, meaning that when functioning normally, they suppress tumor growth. When there is an inherited mutation, these genes produce defective proteins that are less able or unable to check cancer growth.

breast cancer stages—

Stage I means that cancer cells have not spread beyond the breast and the tumor is no more than about 1 inch across. Treated surgically with lumpectomy or mastectomy if desired, and radiation therapy.

Stage II means that cancer has spread to underarm lymph nodes and/or the tumor in the breast is 1 to 2 inches across. Treated surgically with lumpectomy or mastectomy and chemotherapy and radiation therapy.

Stage III, also called locally advanced cancer, means that the tumor in the breast is large (more than 2 inches across), the cancer is extensive in the underarm lymph nodes, or it has spread to other lymph node areas or to other tissues near the breast. Treated with surgery and radiation, as well as chemotherapy, hormonal therapy, or both.

Stage IV is metastatic cancer. The cancer has spread from the breast to other organs of the body. Treated with chemotherapy and/or hormonal therapy to shrink the tumor or destroy cancer cells. Surgery or radiation therapy may be used to control the cancer in the breast, and many women choose to have stem cell transplant.

breast self-examination (BSE)—A technique used by a woman to check her own breasts for lumps and abnormalities.

calcifications—Tiny calcium deposits within the breast, usually detected by mammography. They are a sign of change within the breast and are caused by benign breast conditions or by breast cancer. They are typically monitored by mammograms or biopsy.

cancer suppressor genes—The role of these genes is to suppress tumor growth. Well-known cancer suppressor genes are BRCA1 and BRCA2 genes. When these genes have a mutation, cancer can grow unchecked.

carcinogens—Any substance that causes cancer or promotes cancer growth.

CAT Scan (Computerized axial tomography)—A diagnostic X-ray technique that uses a computer to achieve cross-sectional views of your body, offering a more sensitive and thorough image. CAT scans also deliver a high dose of radiation, so it's generally reserved for use in diagnosing hard to view areas such as bones, brain, liver, or lungs.

chemoprevention—Prevention or reversal of cancer using drugs, chemicals, or other supplements. Tamoxifen is an example of a chemoprevention drug. This is a burgeoning area of research.

chemotherapy—The procedure in which potent cancer-killing drugs are administered to a patient through a pill or intravenously, once every two to three weeks for a period of four to six months. Chemotherapy is considered an adjuvant therapy, meaning it is used in addition to surgery to decrease the chance of a cancer recurring or spreading to other parts of the body. Commonly used chemotherapy drug combinations are CMF (cyclophosphamide, methotrexate, and fluorouracil), CAF (cyclophosphamide, Adriamycin, and fluorouracil), and CA (cyclophosphamide and Adriamycin).

clinical breast exam—The procedure in which a physician manually palpates a woman's breasts for lumps or abnormalities.

cyst—A fluid-filled sac that is usually benign. Cysts sometimes become enlarged before a woman gets her period.

ductal carcinoma in situ (DCIS)—An abnormal finding that is confined to the milk ducts of the breast. It may develop into cancer, but is slow-growing and highly curable.

estrogen—A female sex hormone produced primarily by the ovaries and responsible for menstruation and preparing the body for reproduction. Estrogen is also known to promote growth of some types of breast cancer.

exogenous estrogens—Estrogen not produced by the body, such as those in oral contraceptives or hormone replacement therapy.

false positive—When the result of a test is positive, but later it's discovered that the test was wrong and there was no diseased tissue.

false negative—When the result of a test is negative, but later it's discovered that the test was wrong. For instance, a mammogram finding no suspicious lumps is a false negative if a woman finds her own cancerous lump two months after taking the test.

fibrocystic breast disease—Most doctors no longer use this term, which in the past was a blanket term that described any benign changes in the breast and had been associated with an increased risk of breast cancer. The reality is that some changes in the breasts do not come with an increase in risk, and others do, so doctors have had to be specific about their diagnosis.

first-degree relative—A mother, sister, or daughter.

gene—A segment of DNA, which is the blueprint that carries the complete set of instructions for making all the proteins a cell needs. Each gene contains chemical bases whose formation determines the gene's job and the protein it will produce. Humans have 50,000 to 100,000 genes, which determine characteristics such as eye color, body type, and susceptibility to certain diseases.

genetic counselor—A medical professional who is trained in medical genetics and various aspects of social work and counseling. Counselors come from a variety of specialties, such as nursing, social services, or psychology.

Herceptin—A drug that is FDA-approved for the treatment of breast cancer that has spread beyond the breast and lymph nodes under the arm. Herceptin, a monoclonal antibody, targets a protein that is overproduced by cancer cells in women who have a certain gene mutation called HER2 (human epidermal growth factor receptor 2). A woman can be tested to see if her cancer has excessive amounts of the protein, and if it does, Herceptin may inhibit her tumor growth. Herceptin is reserved for patients who have tried chemotherapy with little success or as a first-line treatment for metastatic disease when used in combination with Taxol.

Hodgkin's disease—a cancer of the lymphatic system that causes a progressive and often fatal enlargement of the lymph nodes, spleen, and general lymphoid tissues. It often begins in the neck and spreads throughout the body.

hormone therapy—This treatment deprives cancer cells of the female hormone estrogen, which some breast cancer cells need to grow. Most patients undergoing hormone therapy are treated with tamoxifen, a known antiestrogen, but other drugs are used as well, such as megestrol, aminoglutethimide, and androgens. In some cases, surgical removal of the ovaries is performed, since the ovaries are where estrogen is manufactured.

hyperplasia—An abnormal increase in the number of cells. This is not harmful unless the cells are irregular. (See atypical hyperplasia)

in situ cancer—The phrase *in situ* means literally *in the site of*. This means that a cancer has not invaded surrounding tissue.

informed consent—The process of informing a patient of all the risks and complications of a procedure, and a patient agreeing to do the procedure in spite of the risks.

IV—The acronym for intravenous, or using a needle inserted into a vein to deliver medications or fluids.

lobular carcinoma in situ (LCIS)—An abnormal finding in the milk-producing glands (lobules) of the breast. LCIS almost never progresses to cancer, although having LCIS does increase your risk of developing breast cancer.

lump—Any kind of mass in the breast or elsewhere in the body.

lumpectomy—Breast-conserving surgery to remove only the malignant lump and a small amount of the surrounding healthy tissue.

lymph node—Small clumps of lymphatic tissue, shaped like a bean, and located throughout the body. They are essential in fighting infection. Lymph nodes in the underarm or chest are a common site for breast cancer to spread. Some nodes are usually removed during a mastectomy or lumpectomy to determine whether they contain cancer cells. If cancer is found, the woman is said to be "node positive" and her cancer is considered more advanced.

lymphedema—When lymph nodes are removed, there is a small risk of lymphedema, or the swelling in the arm caused by excess fluid that collects after surgery. This condition often remains indefinitely.

lymphoma—A cancer that originates in lymph nodes (different from breast cancer that spreads to lymph nodes). The two main types of lymphomas are Hodgkin's disease and non-Hodgkin's lymphoma.

malignant—Containing cancerous cells.

mammography—A low-dose X ray specially designed to detect cancers of the breast. Typically, mammography consists of two X rays of each breast. A mammogram can show a developing tumor before it is large enough to be felt by a woman or her doctor.

margins—The tissue surrounding a cancer. If the margins are clear, the surrounding tissue that was removed with the lump had no sign of errant cancerous cells.

mastectomy—Surgery to remove all or part of the breast.

modified radical mastectomy—Surgery to remove the nipple and surrounding skin, breast tissue, fat and connective tissue, most of the axillary (underarm) lymph nodes and the lining over the chest muscles, but usually leaving the chest muscles intact.

bilateral mastectomy—Surgical removal of both breasts.

menarche—A woman's first menstrual period.

menopause—The time when menstruation ceases and levels of estrogen produced by the ovaries drop dramatically. For most women, menopause occurs in the late forties or early fifties.

meta-analysis—A scientific review of many large-scale studies. These are typically undertaken to increase the population size of studies to gain more accurate assessments of potential risk factors.

metastasis—The spread of cancer from the original site to other parts of the body, such as the liver, bones, or brain. Cancer is typically spread through the lymphatic system or bloodstream.

morphine—Prescription pain-relieving medication often used for pain management during breast cancer treatment.

MRI (magnetic resonance imaging)—An imaging technique that uses a magnet to transmit radio waves through the body. MRI's deliver computerized cross-sectional images of the body onto a computer screen.

mutation—A change in a gene, the subunit of DNA. The mutation causes that gene to malfunction. Changes occur in the order of the chemical bases that make up the coding for a gene. (See gene)

needle biopsy—Removal of a cylinder of tissue or fluid from a lump with a needle and syringe. The needle is inserted into the lump (often with the help of an ultrasound image) and a syringe is used to draw out cells to analyze.

oncologist—A physician who specializes in the diagnosis and treatment of cancer. There are various subspecialties in the field of oncology. Medical oncologists specialize in chemotherapy and other drugs to treat cancer. Radiation oncologists specialize in radiation therapy. Surgical oncologists perform surgery to treat cancer.

oncology social worker—A person with a master's degree in social work who specializes in working with cancer patients.

prophylactic mastectomy—A controversial procedure, sometimes chosen by a woman at high risk of developing cancer, in which both breasts are removed preventively. It also refers to surgery of a healthy breast in a woman who has had breast cancer in the other breast.

prophylactic oophorectomy—Surgical removal of the ovaries preventively in order to reduce the risk of ovarian cancer.

radiation therapy—The use of high-energy X rays to treat cancer. Typically, a woman receives daily radiation treatments for a period of three to six weeks.

raloxifene—An antiestrogenic drug being tested for the prevention of breast cancer.

reconstruction—Surgery done to recreate the breast's shape after a breast has been removed. This procedure can be done at the same time as a mastectomy or sometime in the future.

recurrence—Reappearance of cancer after treatment, at the same site, near the site, or in other areas of the body.

remission—Complete or partial disappearance of the cancer in response to treatment.

risk factor—Anything that increases a person's chance of getting a disease.

second-degree relatives—Aunts, grandmothers, nieces, cousins, or grandchildren.

stem cell transplant—A procedure (previously called *bone marrow transplant*) used when breast cancer is advanced or has recurred as a way of delivering extremely high doses of chemotherapy to the patient. High-dose chemotherapy can severely damage or destroy the patient's bone marrow, the spongy material found inside bones that produces the body's white and red blood cells and platelets. This marrow contains the stem cells that can reproduce all the types of blood cells. In the procedure, stem cells are removed from the blood. The patient is given several high doses of chemotherapy to kill any existing cancer cells as well as the remaining bone marrow. During this time, the patient's immune system is terribly compromised. The healthy stem cells are returned to the body and begin to produce the blood cells the patient needs to survive. Typically, a patient has to stay in the hospital or in an isolated hotel room for a month, until her immune system is strong enough to fight off everyday germs. Stem cell transplants have not been scientifically proven to be more effective than conventional therapies in treating breast cancer. It is a risky procedure that can cause serious side effects and involves a lengthy and expensive hospital stay that may not be covered by the patient's health insurance.

tamoxifen—A type of hormone treatment used to treat breast cancer and to prevent cancer. This drug, an antiestrogen, works against breast cancer in part by attaching to the estrogen receptors of cancerous cells in the breast and blocking out estrogen. Without estrogen, the cancer cells don't seem to thrive.

Taxol—A drug extracted from the bark of the Pacific yew tree. It is used for treating certain women who have advanced breast or ovarian cancer.

ventilator—A machine that is inserted into a critically ill patient's throat and mechanically assists patients in the exchange of oxygen and carbon dioxide.

BIBLIOGRAPHY

American Cancer Society. *Cancer and Genetics.* Huntington, NY: PRI, 1997.

Baider, Lea, Cary L. Cooper, and Atara Kaplan De-Nour. *Cancer and the Family.* West Sussex, England: John Wiley & Sons, 1996.

Bassoff, Evelyn. *Mothering Ourselves.* New York: NAL-Dutton, 1992.

————. *Mothers and Daughters.* New York: Plume, 1988.

Chernin, Kim. *In My Mother's House.* New York: HarperCollins, 1984.

Edelman, Hope. *Motherless Daughters.* New York: Addison-Wesley, 1994.

Feldman, Gayle. *You Don't Have to Be Your Mother.* New York: W. W. Norton, 1994.

Friday, Nancy. *My Mother, My Self.* New York: Dell, 1987.

Kaye, Ronnie. *Spinning Straw into Gold.* New York: Simon & Schuster, 1991.

Kelly, Patricia T. *Understanding Breast Cancer Risk.* Philadelphia: Temple University Press, 1991.

Lorde, Audre. *The Cancer Journals.* San Francisco: Aunt Lute Books, 1980.

Love, Susan. *Dr. Susan Love's Breast Book.* New York: Addison-Wesley, 1995.

Lowinsky, Naomi Ruth. *The Motherline.* Los Angeles: Tarcher, 1993.

————. *Stories from the Motherline.* Los Angeles: Tarcher, 1992.

McCarthy, Peggy, and Jo An Loren, eds. *Breast Cancer? Let Me Check My Schedule.* Boulder, CO: Westview Press, 1997.

Moch, Susan Diemert. *Breast Cancer: Twenty Women's Stories.* New York: NLN, 1995.

National Cancer Institute. *Taking Time: Support for People with Cancer and the People Who Care about Them.* Bethesda, MD: NCI, 1997.

Offit, Kenneth. *Clinical Cancer Genetics.* New York: John Wiley & Sons, 1998.

Quindlen, Anna. *One True Thing.* New York: Bantam Doubleday Dell, 1997.

Pedersen, Lucille. *Breast Cancer: A Family Survival Guide.* Bergin & Garvey, 1995.

Phillips, Shelley. *Beyond the Myths: Mother-Daughter Relationships in Psychology, History, Literature, and Everyday Life.* London: Penguin, 1991.

Rich, Adrienne. *Of Woman Born.* New York: Norton, 1986.

Rollin, Betty. *First You Cry.* New York: Harper, 1976.

Royak-Schaler, Renee, and Beryl Lieff Benderly. *Challenging the Breast Cancer Legacy.* New York, HarperCollins, 1992.

Wadler, Joyce. *My Breast.* New York: Addison-Wesley, 1992.

Waldholz, Michael. *Curing Cancer.* New York: Simon & Schuster, 1997.

Weiss, Robert S. *Learning from Strangers.* New York: Free Press, 1994.

Williams, Terry Tempest. *Refuge: An Unnatural History of Family and Place.* New York: Vintage Books, 1992.

Wittman, Juliet. *Breast Cancer Journal.* Golden, CO: Fulcrum, 1993.